How to Manage and Survive during a Global Crisis

Sharma and Leung explore the differences in the national and organizational responses to COVID-19 across various countries.

The COVID-19 global pandemic is possibly the worst healthcare disaster ever, and recent studies highlight several differences in the response to COVID-19. Some countries acted quickly with strict measures to successfully contain the initial spread of the COVID-19 and minimize the number of cases and deaths, while others have not been as proactive and have suffered more as a result. The book is organized under distinct themes based on the stages of the COVID-19 pandemic, consisting of (a) discovery and early response, (b) global spread and reactions, (c) early successes and failures, and (d) subsequent waves and new strains. It goes on to analyze the differences in national responses to draw important lessons for managers and governments and concludes with policy recommendations.

A useful guide for students, managers, and the general public who are interested in learning about the COVID-19 experience and how such global crises could be managed more effectively in future.

Piyush Sharma is John Curtin Distinguished Professor at Curtin University, Australia. His multidisciplinary research appears in the *Journal of International Business Studies, Journal of the Academy of Marketing Science, Journal of Service Research, International Journal of Research in Marketing*, and *Journal of Business Research*, among others.

Tak Yan Leung is an Associate Professor of Accounting at the University of the Sunshine Coast, Australia. Her research on corporate finance, corporate governance, and executive compensation appears in the *Academy of Management Journal, British Journal of Management, Journal of Business Research, Journal of Corporate Finance, Journal of Economic Behavior and Organization*, and *International Business Review*.

Routledge Advances in Management and Business Studies

Responsible Management and Sustainable Consumption
Creating a Consumer and Enterprise Social Responsibility Index
Edited by Piotr Wachowiak, Anna Dąbrowska, Monika Zajkowska and Celina Sołek-Borowska

Co-operative and Mutual Enterprises Research
A Comprehensive Overview
Tim Mazzarol

Corruption and the Management of Public Safety
The Governance of Technological Systems
Simon Ashley Bennett

Hofstede Matters
Edited by Sławomir Magala, Christiane Erten, Roger Matthew Bell, Marie-Therese Claes, Senem Yazici and Atila Karabag

Entrepreneurship Education and Internationalisation
Cases, Collaborations and Contexts
Edited by Robert James Crammond and Denis Hyams-Ssekasi

Sustainable Business in the Era of Digital Transformation
Strategic and Entrepreneurial Perspectives
Mariusz Sołtysik, Magdalena Wojnarowska, Maria Urbaniec, Vesna Zabkar, Marek Ćwiklicki and Erica Varese

How to Manage and Survive during a Global Crisis
Lessons for Managers from the COVID-19 Pandemic
Piyush Sharma and Tak Yan Leung

For more information about this series, please visit: www.routledge.com/
Routledge-Advances-in-Management-and-Business-Studies/book-series/SE0305

How to Manage and Survive during a Global Crisis

Lessons for Managers from the COVID-19 Pandemic

Piyush Sharma and Tak Yan Leung

Routledge
Taylor & Francis Group

LONDON AND NEW YORK

First published 2025
by Routledge
4 Park Square, Milton Park, Abingdon, Oxon, OX14 4RN

and by Routledge
605 Third Avenue, New York, NY 10158

Routledge is an imprint of the Taylor & Francis Group, an informa business

British Library Cataloguing-in-Publication Data
A catalogue record for this book is available from the British Library

ISBN: 9781032129778 (hbk)
ISBN: 9781032129785 (pbk)
ISBN: 9781003227113 (ebk)

DOI: 10.4324/9781003227113

Typeset in Galliard
by KnowledgeWorks Global Ltd.

Contents

Introduction   1

1 COVID-19 discovery and early response: Unveiling a global crisis   4

2 COVID-19 global spread and reactions: Unity in diversity   20

3 COVID-19 early successes and failures: Battling the unknown   43

4 COVID-19 subsequent waves and new strains: Living with the enemy   59

5 COVID-19 differences in national responses: Different strokes   71

6 COVID-19 business response: Adaptation, resilience, and innovation   89

7 COVID-19 important management lessons: Learning from failures   105

8 Conclusion and recommendations   123

References   *143*
Appendix-I: Country-wise first COVID-19 cases   *163*
Appendix-II: Country-wise early response to COVID-19   *172*

Mini-case I: Samsung response to COVID-19   178
Mini-case II: Digital payments revolution in India   181
Mini-case III: JobKeeper Payment program in Australia   184
Mini-case IV: COVID-19 vaccine diplomacy: The Indian
  experience   187
Index   191

Introduction

Many events in human history have reshaped the course of societies and humanity, challenged the very foundations of our existence, and forced us to redefine our understanding of basic human traits of resilience, adaptability, and leadership in the face of adversity, disasters, and destruction. The COVID-19 pandemic (simply referred to as COVID-19 in the rest of this book for parsimony) is a stark example of such events. From the moment the virus emerged on the global stage, it thrust humanity into an unprecedented crisis, affecting every facet of life, indiscriminately killing vulnerable people, disrupting economies, and testing the mettle of leaders at all levels (Sharma et al., 2020). As a result, COVID-19 is possibly the worst healthcare disaster ever, with about 800 million cases and 7 million deaths reported till 31 August 2023, led by the United States and China, followed by India, France, Germany, and Brazil (WHO, 2023).

Beyond its direct health implications, COVID-19 also unleashed a series of negative socio-economic impacts that disrupted lives, economies, and societies on a global scale (Sharma et al., 2020). COVID-19 also had a devastating economic impact sending shock waves through the world economy and triggering the largest global economic crisis seen in more than a century, with especially severe outcomes in the emerging economies. Global poverty increased for the first time in a generation and unemployment rates rose to levels only seen during the great depression and the two world wars. Disproportionate income losses among disadvantaged populations in particular led to a dramatic rise in socio-economic inequality within and across countries. Most governments around the world responded to the onset of the pandemic with large stimulus programs that were successful at mitigating the worst human costs in the short run. However, this emergency response also exacerbated a number of pre-existing economic fragilities that might pose an obstacle to an equitable recovery.

As the world grappled with the immediate implications of the pandemic, managers found themselves in uncharted waters with no clear idea about how serious this threat to their businesses was and how long it was going to last. Businesses faced unprecedented challenges as they navigated through

DOI: 10.4324/9781003227113-1

economic and environmental uncertainties, government-imposed restrictions such as lockdowns, supply chain disruptions, and remote work dynamics. The swift and drastic changes required a new breed of leadership, not only strategic and visionary but also empathetic, agile, and forward-thinking. Recent studies highlight several differences in the response to COVID-19, with some countries acting quickly with strict measures, such as lockdowns and border closures, to successfully contain its initial spread and minimize the number of cases and deaths (e.g., Australia, New Zealand, Taiwan, and Vietnam) but others have not been as proactive and suffered more as a result (e.g., Italy, Spain, UK, and USA).

Beyond its immediate health impact, COVID-19 illuminated a tapestry of lessons that extend far beyond healthcare systems. It illuminated the indispensable qualities of adaptability, innovation, communication, and empathy – core pillars that every manager should embody when steering their organizations through tumultuous times. In this book, we describe the real-world stories of businesses that weathered the storm and some that faltered in the face of adversity. We delve into the principles of crisis leadership, drawing insights from industries ranging from technology to healthcare, and from countries around the globe. This book is a compendium of knowledge distilled from the collective experience of managers who found ingenious solutions, demonstrated unwavering resolve, and emerged stronger on the other side.

This book is organized into distinct themes based on the stages of COVID-19, consisting of (a) discovery and early response, (b) global spread and reactions, (c) early successes and failures, (d) subsequent waves and new strains. We also analyze the differences in national and organizational responses to draw important lessons for managers and governments followed by our conclusions and recommendations. We use a number of tables, charts, examples, and case studies to explain our results and their implications. This book will be relevant for students and managers to learn from the COVID-19 experience and how to manage such global crises more effectively in future. This book is different from other books on COVID-19 in terms of being more research-focused and evidence-based from a business point of view rather than a healthcare or epidemiological perspective.

We begin this book with an introduction to COVID-19 followed by Chapter 1 to describe its discovery and early response from governments, businesses, consumers, and other organizations around the world. This is followed by a description of the reactions to the rapid global spread of COVID-19 in Chapter 2. Next, we review the early successes and failures in dealing with COVID-19 in Chapter 3. Chapter 4 looks at the challenges faced in dealing with the subsequent waves and new strains of COVID-19 and Chapter 5 documents the differences in national responses to COVID-19. Next, we describe the business response to COVID-19 (adaptation, resilience, and innovation) in Chapter 6 and draw important lessons from the successes and failures of the global response to COVID-19 in Chapter 7. Finally, we conclude with Chapter 8 describing our conclusion and recommendations for managers in dealing with similar global crises in the future based on learnings from COVID-19 global pandemic.

Each chapter will illuminate a specific facet of crisis management, from transforming remote work into a competitive advantage to building resilient supply chains, fostering employee well-being, and embracing digital transformation, we uncover a roadmap that guides managers through uncharted territory. More than a survival guide, this book is a call to action – a testament to the resilience of human spirit and the transformative power of leadership. It beckons managers, both seasoned and emerging, to rise to the occasion, embrace challenges as opportunities, and lead with empathy, innovation, and the unwavering belief that even amidst chaos, clarity can be found, and success can be redefined.

1 COVID-19 discovery and early response

Unveiling a global crisis

1.1 Introduction

In December 2019, a cluster of pneumonia cases of unknown origin emerged in Wuhan, China (Shereen et al., 2020). Medical professionals in the city observed a pattern of respiratory illness among patients with links to a seafood market. The causative agent was identified as a novel coronavirus, initially termed 2019-nCoV. Chinese authorities acted swiftly, isolating the virus's genetic sequence and sharing it globally. This information was crucial for the rapid development of diagnostic tests and potential treatments. By January 2020, the virus was officially named SARS-CoV-2 due to its genetic similarity to the severe acute respiratory syndrome (SARS) virus (Donthu & Gustafsson, 2020; Sharma et al., 2020).

China's initial response involved strict containment measures, including lockdowns, travel restrictions, and quarantine of affected areas (Allel et al., 2020). As the virus spread beyond China's borders, nations worldwide faced the challenge of managing its rapid transmission. The World Health Organization (WHO) declared coronavirus disease 2019 (COVID-19) a Public Health Emergency of International Concern on 30 January 2020, urging countries to prepare for potential outbreaks. Many nations implemented early measures, including travel advisories, screening at airports, and quarantine protocols. However, the virus's highly contagious nature presented difficulties in containment. By March 2020, the WHO declared COVID-19 a pandemic, highlighting the global scale of the crisis (WHO, 2020).

The early response to COVID-19 was marked by several challenges. Limited understanding of the virus led to evolving guidelines and recommendations. The shortage of personal protective equipment (PPE), testing kits, and medical resources strained healthcare systems globally. Additionally, the interconnectedness of our world facilitated rapid international spread, testing the effectiveness of early containment efforts. Communication hurdles and misinformation further complicated the response. Governments and health organizations struggled to disseminate accurate information amidst a flood of rumors and false claims, leading to confusion among the public. We begin this chapter by identifying the multifaceted adverse impact of COVID-19 on

DOI: 10.4324/9781003227113-2

public health, economic activity, and output, businesses and consumers, education, transportation, mental well-being, social cohesion, etc.

COVID-19 soon became one of the most significant public health crises of our time. It has exposed vulnerabilities in healthcare systems, challenged governments, and altered the way we live and interact with the world (Hartley & Perencevich, 2020). The virus led to millions of deaths and caused immense suffering among those infected as healthcare systems in many countries struggled to cope with the overwhelming demand for medical services (The Lancet Public Health, 2022), which in turn resulted in shortages of essential supplies, stretched medical personnel, and overwhelmed hospital facilities (Hartley & Perencevich, 2020). The pandemic exposed the vulnerabilities and inequalities in global healthcare systems, underlining the urgent need for improved preparedness and equitable access to healthcare (Hobin & Smith, 2020). Next, we describe some unique characteristics of COVID-19 that made it such a huge challenge for people, organizations, and governments around the world.

1.2   Global scale of COVID-19 pandemic

COVID-19 swiftly transcended borders, becoming a global pandemic within months of its emergence in late 2019, affecting virtually every country, spanning continents, and impacting diverse populations (Lee, 2020; MacIntyre, 2020). Figure 1.1 shows the rapid country-wise spread of COVID-19 during the first six months from the discovery of the first positive case, based on the visualization of data available from the WHO COVID-19 database.

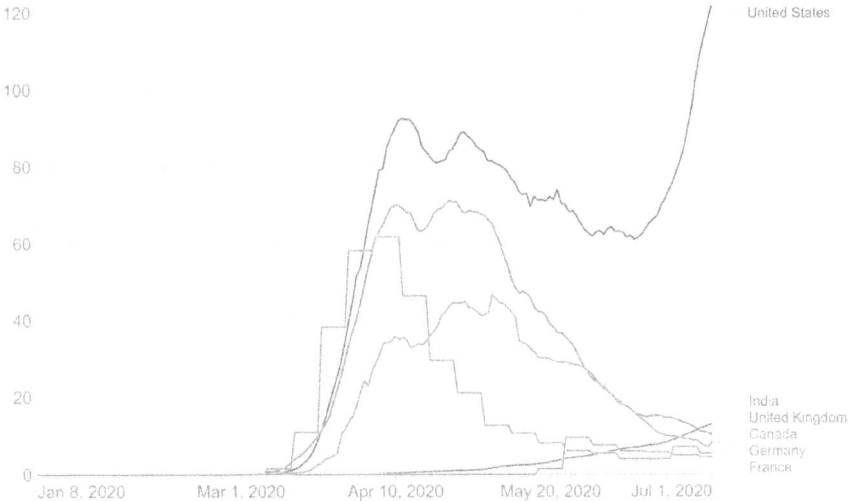

Figure 1.1 Daily new confirmed COVID-19 cases per million people (first six months, seven-days rolling average)

Source: WHO COVID-19 Dashboard

1.2.1   *Overwhelmed healthcare systems*

COVID-19 placed immense strain on healthcare systems worldwide (Tulenko & Vervoort, 2020). Hospitals became overwhelmed with COVID-19 patients, leading to shortages of critical medical supplies, ventilators, and healthcare personnel (Kirk & Mitchell, 2023). The crisis forced healthcare professionals to make difficult decisions about resource allocation and patient care, such as emergency department and outpatient waiting times, delayed elective surgery, and intensive care unit (ICU) refusals. Staff fatigue and burnout were also probably exacerbated by the pandemic, although their broader impact on patient outcomes is unknown. Figure 1.2 shows the key challenges faced by healthcare systems and their ability to cope with COVID-19.

Theme	Challenges	Example
Financial Impact	• Care delays and cancellations disrupted revenue streams and severely affected provider finances • Providers incurred many pandemic-related costs (and paid premiums) to purchase supplies and restructure clinical workflows	• Financial losses for hospitals between March 2020 and June 2020 are estimated to exceed $200 billion • The cost of refilling essential medicines increased by 62% during April 2020
Supply Chain	• Health systems across the country reported persistent shortages of PPE, essential medicines, and medical devices • Outsourced manufacturing and depleted domestic reserves contributed to supply chain vulnerabilities	• Hospital demand for dexamethasone increased by 610% while fill rates declined to 54% • Over 20% of nursing homes nationwide reported severe PPE shortages well into the summer of 2020
Workforce	• Pre-pandemic staffing shortages were an obstacle to the development of surge capacity for COVID-19 • COVID-19 has exacerbated the existing challenges of burnout among health professionals	• Staff shortages for critical care led to increased demand among health systems for temporary clinicians • Surveys of providers indicated elevated levels of stress and symptoms of anxiety, depression, and post-traumatic stress
System and Community-Wide Coordination	• Coordination within health systems and with other sectors was complicated by decentralized governance models • Outdated technical infrastructure created challenges for data sharing	• Health department capacity varied widely across the country, requiring health systems in rural and underserved areas to take on additional responsibilities • Funding for the Hospital Preparedness Program was reduced by 46% between 2003 and 2020, limiting the resources available to hospitals to coordinate emergency response

Figure 1.2 Challenges faced by healthcare systems during COVID-19

Source: National Academy of Medicine, USA (Balser et al., 2021)

1.2.2 Large-scale loss of life

COVID-19 has led to a significant loss of life with millions of people succumbing to the virus, leaving a trail of grief and bereavement for families and communities (Simonsen & Viboud, 2021). The toll on vulnerable populations, including the elderly and those with underlying health conditions, has been particularly devastating. Figure 1.3A shows the trend in the total number of deaths (seven-days rolling average) due to COVID-19 until 30 June 2022.

Countries around the world used different methods to test and report COVID-19 deaths, which has made the comparison of death tolls and other health outcomes of COVID-19 quite difficult. To overcome these challenges, many countries have turned to excess mortality as a more accurate measure of the true impact of the pandemic. Excess mortality is defined as the difference in the total number of deaths in a crisis compared to those expected under normal conditions. COVID-19 excess mortality accounts for both the total number of deaths directly attributed to the virus and its indirect impact, including disruption to essential health services or travel schedules. Figure 1.3B shows the excess mortality trends during COVID-19.

1.2.3 Devastating economic impact

COVID-19 triggered severe economic repercussions, widespread job losses, business closures, and economic recessions around the world (Sharma et al., 2020). The economic fallout has had far-reaching effects on individuals' livelihoods and well-being. For example, global gross domestic product (GDP) fell by 3.4% in 2020, which translates to more than two trillion US dollars of lost

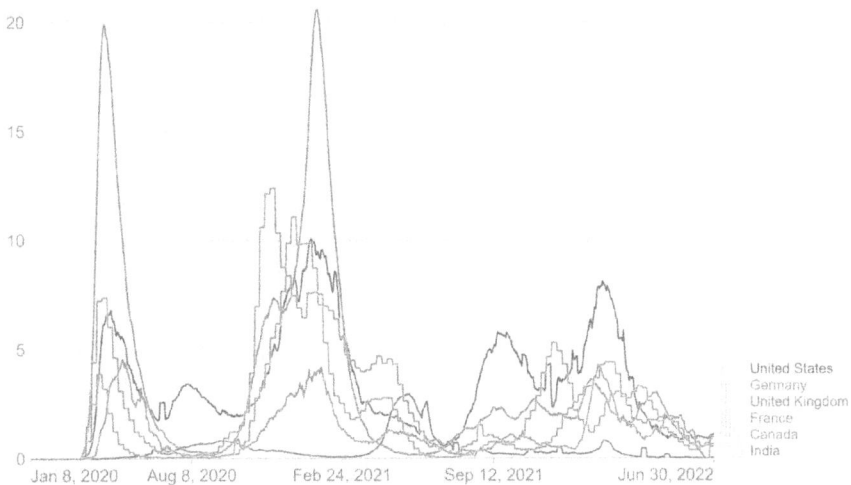

Figure 1.3A Daily new confirmed COVID-19 deaths per million people
Source: WHO COVID-19 Dashboard

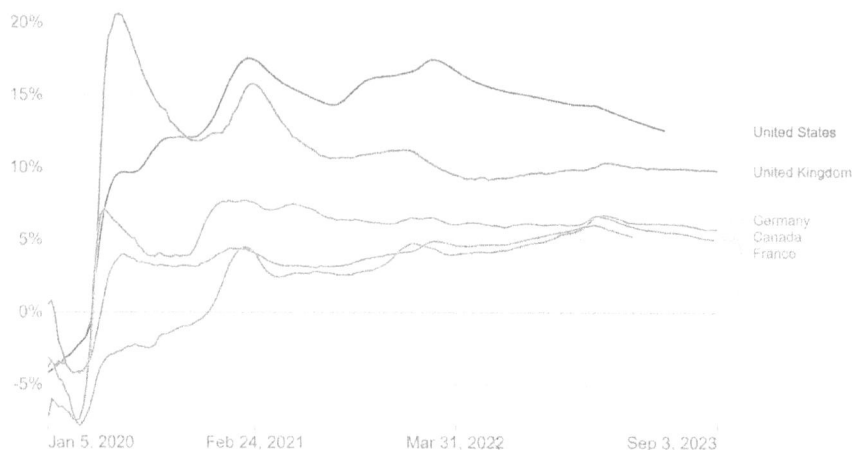

Figure 1.3B Excess mortality: Cumulative deaths vs. projections (%)
Source: WHO COVID-19 Dashboard

economic output based on the 84.9 trillion US dollars global GDP in 2020 (Statista, 2023). Similarly, the global unemployment rate rose to 5.77% and the global goods trade volume declined by 12.9% in April 2020. However, the global economy recovered quickly after the initial shock and reached positive growth again in 2021, with 96.3 trillion US dollars in global GDP and registered a further 3.0% growth in 2022, despite the outbreak of ongoing war between Russia and Ukraine since February 2022. Figure 1.4A shows the loss

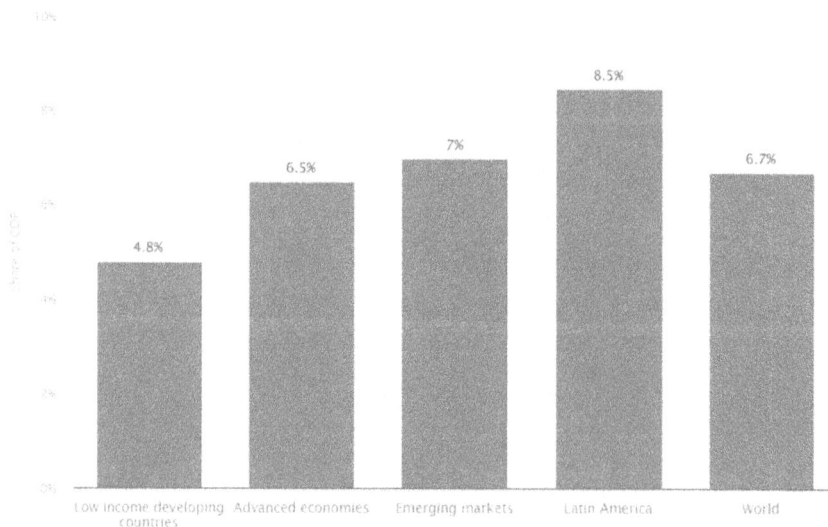

Figure 1.4A Share of GDP loss due to COVID-19 in 2020
Source: Statista.com (2023)

of GDP based on economic growth or status and the world as a whole. As we can see, the worst economic impact was experienced by the Latin American countries (−8.5%), followed by the emerging markets (−7%), and advanced economies (−6.5%), whereas the low-income developing countries suffered less (−4.8%) probably due to their relative disconnect from the global economy, and thus less exposure to the vagaries of global economic events.

The short-term government responses to the pandemic were very quick in most developed countries and much slower in less developed countries, as expected (World Bank, 2023). Governments deployed many policy tools, including direct income support measures, debt freezes, and asset purchase programs by central banks, many of which were totally unprecedented or never implemented at such a large scale. As shown in Figure 1.4B, these fiscal initiatives varied in size and scope based on the ability and willingness of governments to spend on support programs. For example, the fiscal response as a share of the GDP was large in high-income countries, mixed in middle-income countries, and very low to non-existent in low-income countries, possibly due to their limited access to credit markets and high levels of pre-existing government debt. All these fiscal responses also had many negative outcomes, including an increase in nonperforming loans, delayed resolution of distressed loans,

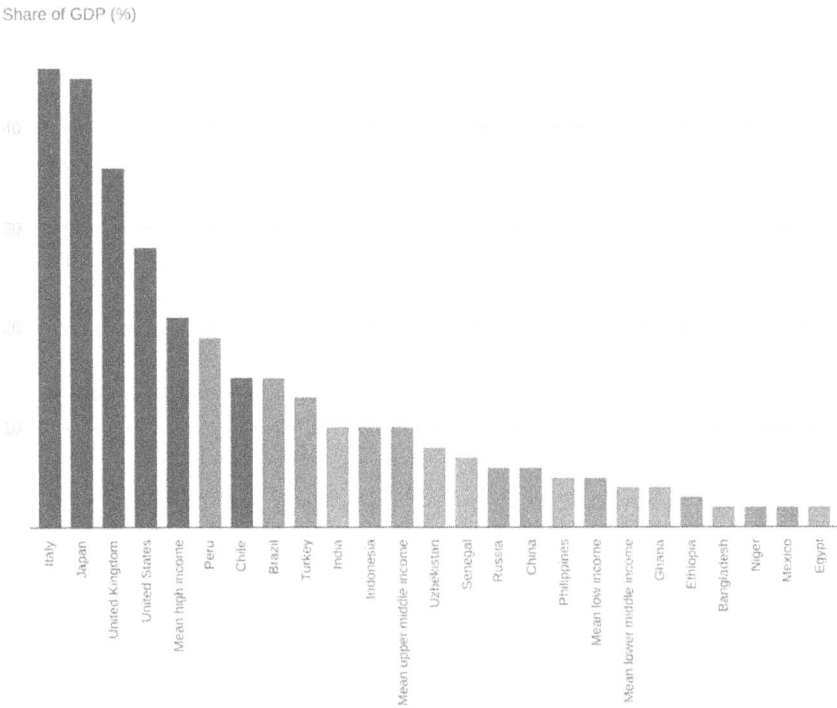

Figure 1.4B Fiscal responses to COVID-19 (as % share of GDP)
Source: World Development Report 2022 (World Bank, 2023)

tighter access to credit, and higher levels of sovereign debt, which need to be addressed in a proactive manner to free up fiscal resources needed to support the recovery.

In fact, even the combination of policies that were used to combat the short-term economic impact of COVID-19, differed greatly across countries, based on the availability of resources and the specific nature of risks faced by each country (World Bank, 2023). As shown in Figure 1.4C, besides direct income support programs, many governments and central banks also used specific policies to provide temporary debt relief, such as freeze on debt repayments for household mortgages and business loans. Interestingly, while these programs helped mitigate the immediate short-term liquidity crisis faced by households and businesses, these may have also unwittingly led to glossing over the actual financial conditions of the borrowers, thus creating a lack of transparency about the real extent and nature of credit risk and overall health of many economies around the world. As discussed earlier, governments around the world need to deal with these issues very urgently.

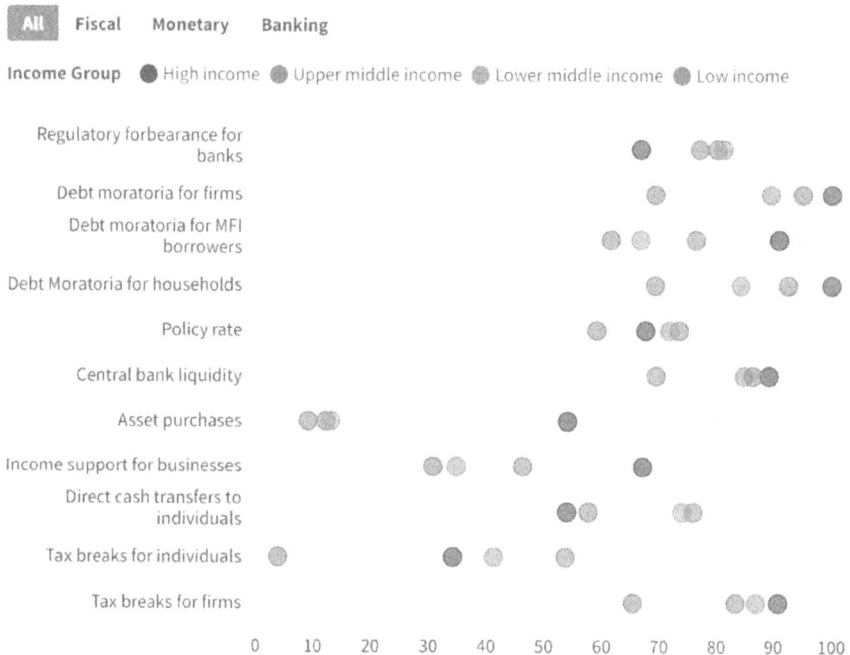

Figure 1.4C Diverse policy responses to COVID-19

Source: World Development Report 2022 (World Bank, 2023)

1.2.4 *Mental health crisis*

The pandemic precipitated a parallel mental health crisis, with rising rates of anxiety, depression, and other psychological challenges due to the isolation imposed by lockdowns and the fear of infection took a toll on mental well-being. A report by Headspace (2020) shows that almost three-quarters (74%) of the young participants in its study felt a little (47%) or a lot worse (27%), with most of them (86%) reporting a negative impact on their mood (75%), well-being, or sleep (59%) during COVID-19. Similarly, most of them (90%) also reported a negative effect on their physical activities and exercise (55%) and regular routine (75%). Seventy-seven percent of young people reported a negative impact on some aspects of their relationships, especially their relationships with friends (70%). Seventy-seven percent of young people reported a negative impact on either their work or financial situation (61%) and studies (65%). Finally, only about half (45%) reported a negative effect on their home and living situation, compared to other aspects of their lives, which probably highlights the important role played by families during COVID-19. Figure 1.5 shows a similar negative impact of COVID-19 on key mental health indicators in the adult US population, including symptoms related to anxiety and/ or depressive disorder (Panchal et al., 2023).

Mental health service providers have tried to cope with the disruptions caused by COVID-19, by delivering their services through alternative channels, such as online appointments and contact-less deliveries, using community-based initiatives for faster adaptation and provision of psychosocial support to those who need it the most (WHO, 2022). International organizations have also provided the necessary tools and resources to help first responders, public health planners, and the general public deal with this unprecedented crisis. In particular, WHO has recommended that countries may adopt the following approaches to deal with the adverse mental health consequences of COVID-19:

- Promote, protect, and care for mental health, including social and financial protection to safeguard people from domestic violence or poverty.
- Communicate widely about COVID-19 to counter misinformation, especially on social media, to minimize its adverse impact on mental health.

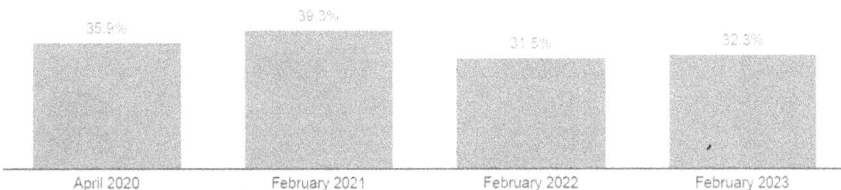

Figure 1.5 Share of adults with symptoms of anxiety/depression during COVID-19

Source: Household Pulse Survey 2020–23, US Census Bureau

- Ensure widespread availability of mental health and psychosocial support facilities by ramping up access to self-help and supporting community-wide initiatives.
- Support recovery from COVID-19 by building mental health services for the future.

1.2.5   Educational disruption

COVID-19 disrupted education on an unprecedented scale with school closures and shift to remote/online learning causing disparities in access to quality education as students, parents, and educators faced challenges in adapting to new learning modalities (Tarkar, 2020). A recent report shows that country-wide school closures as a result of COVID-19 affected 1.5 billion (91.3%) of enrolled students in 191 countries worldwide (UNESCO, 2020). The move to online delivery of education had a particularly severe educational, emotional, and social impact on students from the most socially and financially disadvantaged sections of society (Dorn et al., 2021). The potential negative effects on these students include digital exclusion, poor technology management, greater psychosocial challenges, and long-term educational disengagement (Drane et al., 2020). Besides having to deal with continuing COVID-19 cases even till the end of 2022, schools also faced severe staff shortages, high rates of absenteeism and quarantines, and frequent school closures right through COVID-19 (Kuhfeld et al., 2022). In addition, both students and educators continued to struggle with mental health challenges, higher rates of violence and misbehavior inside and outside the classroom, and concerns about lost instructional time in pandemic (Kuhfeld et al., 2022). In this context, Figure 1.6A shows the key statistics related to the negative impact of COVID-19 on learning gap due to unfinished learning, a key educational outcome.

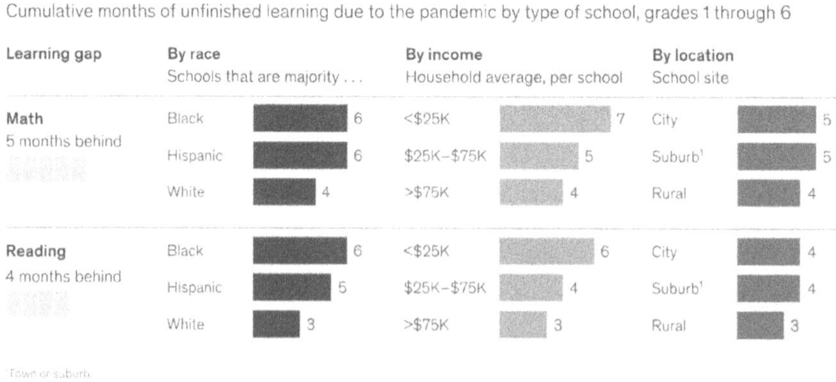

Cumulative months of unfinished learning due to the pandemic by type of school, grades 1 through 6

Learning gap	By race Schools that are majority . . .		By income Household average, per school		By location School site	
Math 5 months behind	Black	6	<$25K	7	City	5
	Hispanic	6	$25K–$75K	5	Suburb[1]	5
	White	4	>$75K	4	Rural	4
Reading 4 months behind	Black	6	<$25K	6	City	4
	Hispanic	5	$25K–$75K	4	Suburb[1]	4
	White	3	>$75K	3	Rural	3

Town or suburb.

Figure 1.6A Negative impact of COVID-19 on education
Source: McKinsey & Company

426–705   128–188   554–893

Existing racial   Incremental increase in   Total
achievement gap   overall achievement
gap due to COVID-19

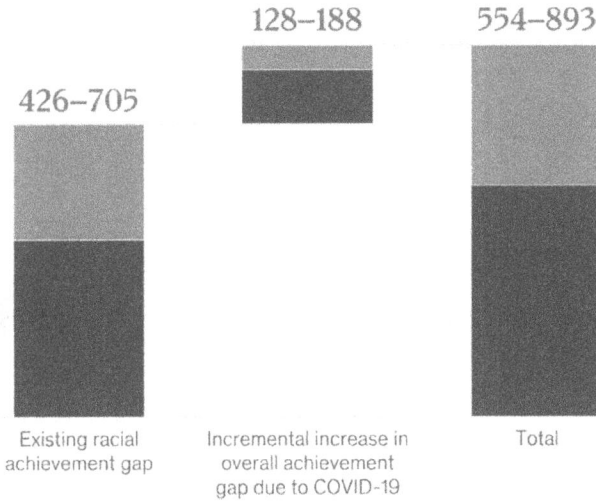

Figure 1.6B Long-term loss of economic potential due to COVID-19 ($billions)
Source: McKinsey & Company

More alarmingly, Figure 1.6B shows the long-term negative impact of COVID-19 on the economic potential of an entire cohort of students due to lost learning potential (billion $ per year), which in turn is expected to further widen the existing racial achievement gap between Whites and Blacks in the USA (Dorn et al., 2021).

1.2.6 Vaccine development and distribution

The COVID-19 crisis spurred an unprecedented global effort to develop and distribute vaccines at an accelerated pace with the vaccination campaigns emerging as a critical public health response to curb the spread of the virus (WHO, 2022). However, there were also many controversies about the development and use of vaccines among people who were concerned about their long-term impact due to the limited testing of these vaccines and uncertainty about their efficacy in preventing the disease or the complications caused by the side effects of their use. More than 30 vaccines have been approved for general or emergency use in countries around the world and over 13 billion doses had been administered worldwide by the end of 2022. However, many countries (e.g., in Africa) have managed to vaccinate only small parts of their populations, and as a result even three years after COVID-19 emerged, almost one-third of the global population is yet to receive a single vaccine dose. Figure 1.7A shows the country-wise share of people with at least one COVID-19 dose by December 2022, and Figure 1.7B shows the COVID-19 vaccine coverage in six major countries, including total number of doses, share of people with at least one dose, complete initial protocol, and booster doses.

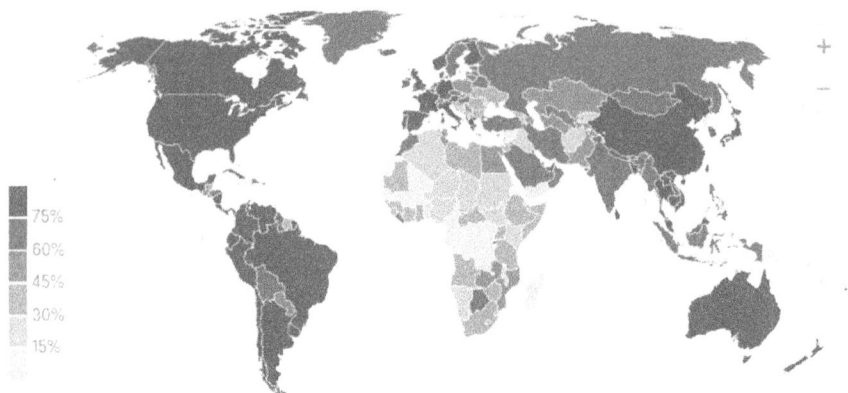

Figure 1.7A Global COVID-19 vaccination divide
Source: Our world in data

1.2.7   *Challenges to healthcare equity*

COVID-19 highlighted disparities in healthcare access and outcomes, disproportionately affecting marginalized communities and underserved populations. For example, vulnerable populations, especially those with lower education and income levels, faced significant obstacles in accessing healthcare services due to a number of factors, including lack of insurance,

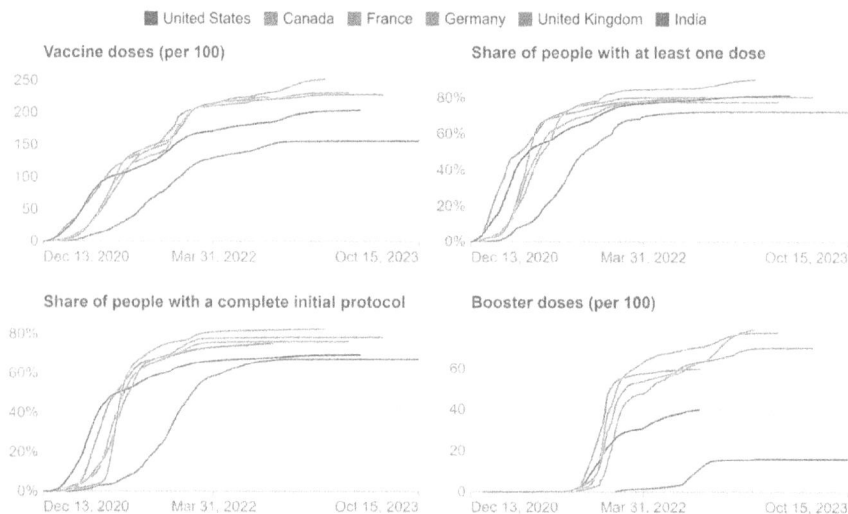

Figure 1.7B COVID-19 vaccine coverage
Source: WHO COVID-19 Dashboard; Our world in data (ourworldindata.org)

transportation issues, or limited availability of healthcare facilities. Racial and ethnic minorities who generally also tend to be economically disadvantaged, were also adversely affected by COVID-19 in a disproportionate manner, with higher rates of infections, hospitalizations, and deaths compared to mainstream populations that are generally more privileged. Socioeconomically disadvantaged populations also often have higher rates of pre-existing health conditions or co-morbidities, such as diabetes, obesity, and hypertension, which are risk factors for severe complications from COVID-19. Many essential workers such as healthcare workers, retail employees, delivery persons, transportation workers, and others who couldn't work from home are often from lower-income backgrounds. As a result, they faced higher risks of exposure to the virus due to the unique nature of their jobs.

Many healthcare facilities and communities in under-served areas with mostly socio-economically disadvantaged communities, faced shortages of PPE and medical resources, which put both healthcare workers and patients at increased risk of infection and death from COVID-19. Marginalized communities, who already face mental health disparities, also experienced heightened stress and mental health challenges during COVID-19, due to isolation, economic stress, and fear of the virus. Even when vaccines became available, vaccine distribution initially faced challenges in ensuring equitable access. Some communities, particularly those with lower trust in healthcare systems, faced vaccine hesitancy. Efforts were made to address these issues through targeted outreach and education but language barriers and limited health literacy posed challenges in understanding and following public health guidelines, which in turn affected people's ability to receive timely and accurate information about the virus.

Socioeconomically disadvantaged people were also more likely to face job loss or financial hardship due to frequent lockdowns and economic downturns during COVID-19, which in turn had a cascading effect on their ability to access food, education, healthcare, housing, and other essential services. The long-term consequences of COVID-19 are still being discovered and we expect that it will have long-lasting effects on healthcare equity, particularly if the existing disparities are not actively addressed. These disparities further underscore the need for health equity in public health responses. Figure 1.8 highlights the eight dimensions of health inequity in the context of COVID-19.

1.2.8   *Collaborative responses despite differences*

Notwithstanding its devastating impact on the global economy and healthcare systems, paradoxically enough, COVID-19 also sparked a new spirit of collaboration and unusual alliances involving governments, public agencies, civic bodies, healthcare companies, manufacturers, retailers, logistics and

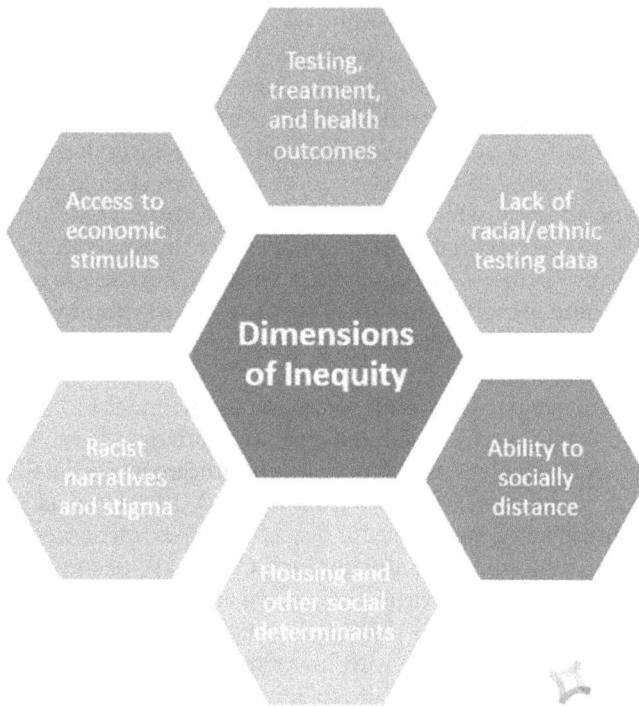

Figure 1.8 COVID-19 and dimensions of health inequity

Source: Health resources in action (www.hria.org)

supply chain providers, and even common citizens around the world (WEF, 2022). Nations and organizations collaborated on an unprecedented scale to share scientific knowledge, coordinate responses, and provide resources to the hardest-hit regions. The crisis prompted a collective effort to find solutions and strategies for mitigation, including the formation of multi-disciplinary and cross-cultural teams to tackle every conceivable aspect of COVID-19 to halt its rapid spread. Collaboration became a constant refrain throughout the pandemic, fueled by global digital connectedness, which facilitated the scientific process, most notably in the rapid vaccine development, a process that would have taken decades under normal circumstances (Bernardo et al., 2021).

All this was possible due to rapid consolidation of global data and statistics about the COVID-19 outbreak and its spread, which in turn triggered the formation of partnerships that would not have been possible otherwise. Bernardo et al. (2021) identified more than 60 projects based on collaboration during COVID-19 and categorized these into five themes, namely artificial intelligence, crowdsourcing, data propagation, hardware design and development, and knowledge dissemination. They highlighted that researchers and citizen scientists struggled to gather high-quality data from an overwhelming amount of information during the early stages of the pandemic. However, with passage of time, more refined and curated datasets emerged, which helped projects using visualizations or models that depended on access to data with consistent and reliable quality. A thread of collaboration weaved throughout the pandemic response, which will shape future efforts by working across boundaries to create better products, processes, and solutions to tackle societal challenges. Exhibit 1.1 shows some examples of such cross-country and multinational collaborative efforts during COVID-19.

Exhibit 1.1 Examples of collaboration during COVID-19

- Crowdsourcing was used as a means to collect and analyze data, help with contact tracing, and scale up the design and production of PPE by sharing the designs for 3D printing (Bernardo et al., 2021).
- Similarly, an international consortium of entrepreneurs and researchers developed a ventilator using an open-source design.
- A coalition of non-government and government organizations, led by White House Office of Science and Technology Policy, created a shared open resource of more than 200,000 research articles on COVID-19 to help worldwide researchers.

1.3 Conclusion

The discovery of COVID-19 and its early response serve as a poignant reminder of the interconnectedness of our world and the challenges that come with emerging infectious diseases. The rapid and collaborative efforts of scientists, healthcare workers, and governments laid the foundation for the fight against the pandemic. As nations continue to grapple with the long-term effects of COVID-19, the lessons learned from its discovery and early response will undoubtedly shape future strategies for pandemic preparedness and global health security. As the public health crisis caused by COVID-19 continues to evolve, with the emergence of new variants and challenges related to vaccine distribution and hesitancy, we need ongoing vigilance and adaptability to navigate the uncertainties of the pandemic's future phases. COVID-19 remains a stark reminder of the profound impact a public health crisis can have on society. It has necessitated rapid responses, innovative solutions, and international cooperation.

1.4 Future lessons for managers

The discovery and early response to COVID-19 highlighted the importance of swift and transparent information sharing between nations. Collaboration and data exchange allowed for a better understanding of the virus and accelerated the development of treatments and vaccines. The pandemic underscored the significance of well-prepared healthcare systems, stockpiles of medical supplies, and efficient testing capabilities. Furthermore, the global response revealed the need for international coordination to mitigate the impact of a rapidly spreading virus. The crisis prompted nations to rethink their approach to pandemic preparedness, emphasizing early detection, data sharing, and community engagement. While the crisis has tested the resilience of healthcare systems and communities, it has also demonstrated the capacity of individuals and organizations to come together in the face of adversity. As the world continues to grapple with COVID-19 and the possibility of having to face and deal with similar pandemics in future, it is a stark reminder of the critical importance of public health infrastructure, preparedness, and global solidarity in addressing complex health challenges (Maani & Galea, 2020).

Based on the early efforts to control COVID-19, it is clear that we need a swift and coordinated response by governments, health organizations, and communities to be able to contain any such global crisis in future. We also need transparent and clear communication from health authorities and governments to build public trust, disseminate accurate information, and ensure compliance with public health measures. Effective control of a global pandemic like COVID-19 also requires international cooperation, information sharing, and resource allocation through effective and selfless collaborations among nations, organizations, and researchers. Similarly, robust plans to face any global crisis should be in place, including surge capacity in healthcare systems, stockpiles of medical supplies, and clear response protocols, to manage such global crises in future more effectively. Widespread testing facilities, effective contact tracing, and isolation measures are fundamental to managing such outbreaks.

We also need to ensure that healthcare systems have the spare capacity to handle any rapid escalation in patient volume without becoming overwhelmed. This includes having sufficient medical staff, hospital beds, ventilators, and other critical resources. Similarly, early implementation and compliance of measures like mask-wearing, social distancing, and hand hygiene can significantly reduce transmission rates. A well-organized and efficient vaccination campaign is essential to achieve herd immunity and prevent future outbreaks besides countering any misinformation or rumor campaigns spread by vested interests. Vulnerable and marginalized communities are often disproportionately affected by pandemics. Efforts to address health disparities and ensure equitable access to healthcare and resources are crucial. Striking a balance between public health measures and the economic impact is a challenging but necessary consideration. In this context, providing economic support for individuals and businesses affected by lockdowns or restrictions is vital.

As the virus continues to mutate, the ability to quickly identify and respond to these variants is crucial to prevent their spread and modify vaccination strategies, as required. Lessons from COVID-19 and the other recent global pandemics, such as the H1N1 influenza pandemic in 2009 or the SARS outbreak in 2003, should be well-documented to help inform preparedness and response efforts. Given the evolving nature of pandemics, responses may need to be adjusted using flexibility in approach, along with the ability to adapt to new information and circumstances. Continued investment in research, development, and innovation is vital for the development of treatments, vaccines, and improved healthcare infrastructure. All these implications highlight the complex and multifaceted nature of pandemic control efforts and serve as important lessons for future preparedness and response efforts to manage the challenges of emerging infectious diseases and other global health crises in future.

2 COVID-19 global spread and reactions

Unity in diversity

2.1 Rapid global spread

COVID-19 showcased the interconnectedness of our modern world. What began as a localized outbreak in Wuhan, China, swiftly evolved into a global pandemic. The virus exploited the ease and speed of international travel, crossing borders with alarming rapidity. By early 2020, numerous countries reported their first cases, marking the virus' successful infiltration of various regions. Figure 2.1 shows the overall figures for confirmed cases, deaths, hospital admissions, and patients in ICU per million people, due to COVID-19.

2.2 Economic disruption

COVID-19's economic impact has been profound and widespread. Lockdowns, travel restrictions, and social distancing measures forced businesses to shut down or operate at limited capacity, leading to massive job losses, business closures, and disruptions in supply chains. The global economy contracted significantly, with various sectors such as tourism, hospitality, and retail being hit hardest. Governments worldwide had to implement stimulus packages and financial aid to mitigate the economic fallout, leading to increased public debt and mixed success in dealing with the pandemic. COVID-19 has inflicted profound economic disruption on a global scale, sending shockwaves through economies, businesses, and people's livelihoods. This description outlines the multifaceted economic impact of the pandemic.

Widespread job losses: COVID-19 led to massive job losses across various sectors, particularly in industries highly susceptible to social distancing restrictions such as hospitality, travel, and entertainment, with layoffs, furloughs, and reduced working hours left millions unemployed or underemployed. As governments implemented strict measures to curb the spread of the virus, such as lockdowns and restrictions on non-essential businesses – these led to closures or reduced operations for a wide range of industries, particularly those reliant on in-person interactions (e.g., hospitality, retail, entertainment). This in turn led to widespread job losses. Similarly, disruptions in global supply chains caused by lockdowns, travel restrictions, and factory closures impacted

DOI: 10.4324/9781003227113-3

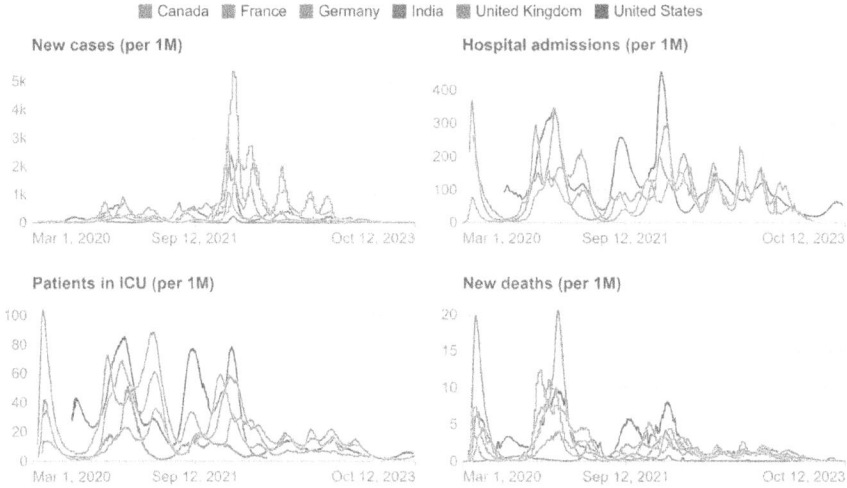

Figure 2.1 Overall figures for COVID-19 impact on health outcomes
Source: WHO COVID-19 Dashboard; Our world in data (ourworldindata.org)

manufacturing and production, – also resulted in significant job cuts in related industries, such as transportation and warehousing.

With people staying home and adhering to social distancing measures, consumer demand for non-essential goods and services also dropped significantly, which resulted in reduced revenue for businesses, such as cinemas, restaurants, hotels, tourist resorts, and shopping malls, which also resulted in many employees being laid-off or put on furlough (leave without pay). The travel and tourism industry was severely affected by the pandemic in particular, with airlines, hotels, cafes, restaurants, retail stores, and other related businesses experiencing a sharp decline in customers. This resulted in a large number of job losses within this sector. Small businesses, which often operate on narrow profit margins, were particularly vulnerable to the economic shocks caused by the pandemic. Many lacked the financial resources to weather extended closures or reduced customer traffic. Entertainment and popular events such as concerts, sports, conferences, and other large gatherings were canceled or severely limited, leading to layoffs in the event planning, hospitality, and entertainment industries. Figure 2.2 shows jobs with high physical proximity that were most severely affected during the pandemic.

COVID-19 also led to a dramatic drop in the demand for oil that resulted in a collapse of global oil prices, which in turn resulted in significant job losses in the oil and gas industry worldwide. While some jobs shifted to remote work, many others could not adapt to this model which led to massive job losses, especially in those industries that require a face-to-face interaction, such as events, construction, transportation, etc. Paradoxically, some businesses accelerated automation efforts to reduce the need for in-person

Overall-physical-proximity score by work arena (based on human interaction and work-environment metrics), score out of 100

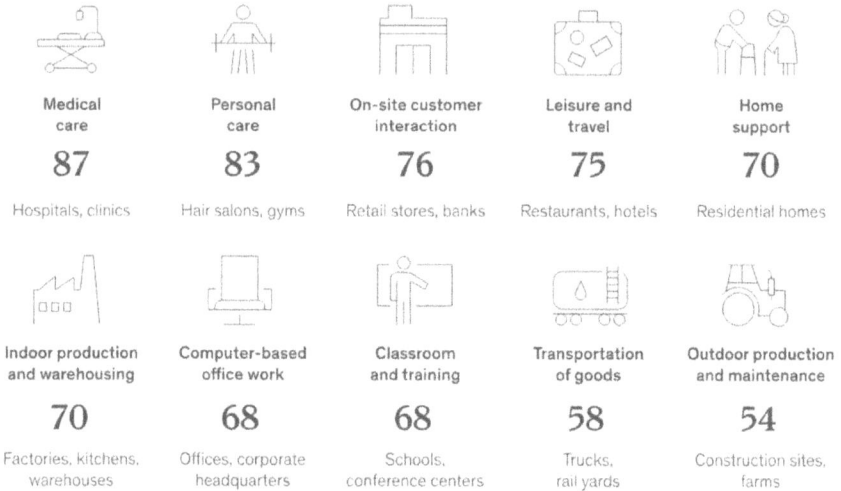

Medical care	Personal care	On-site customer interaction	Leisure and travel	Home support
87	**83**	**76**	**75**	**70**
Hospitals, clinics	Hair salons, gyms	Retail stores, banks	Restaurants, hotels	Residential homes

Indoor production and warehousing	Computer-based office work	Classroom and training	Transportation of goods	Outdoor production and maintenance
70	**68**	**68**	**58**	**54**
Factories, kitchens, warehouses	Offices, corporate headquarters	Schools, conference centers	Trucks, rail yards	Construction sites, farms

Figure 2.2 Jobs with high physical proximity most affected by COVID-19

Source: McKinsey & Company (https://www.mckinsey.com/featured-insights)

labor, which also resulted in fewer jobs, such as online shopping and automated order processing. Similarly, the adoption of more online tutorials and classes in schools and universities resulted in many regular staff members being made redundant or adopting voluntary early retirements around the world, many of whom decided to stay retired and not return to work later (Burki, 2020).

Economic uncertainty caused by the pandemic also led to reduced investment and postponement of expansion plans by many businesses, which also resulted in job cuts. Even when restrictions were lifted, concerns about the virus and the need for safety measures like social distancing and sanitation led to reduced capacity in many businesses, which in turn limited their ability to rehire. Interestingly, frequent and prolonged closures of schools and daycare facilities forced the parents to stay at home to take care of the education and welfare of their children, which meant that many parents could not go to work, and this also affected workforce participation, especially for those with young children. The combined impact of all these factors created an unprecedented economic crisis, with millions of people losing their jobs or facing reduced work hours. Government stimulus measures, unemployment benefits, and support programs were implemented in many developed countries to help mitigate the economic fallout of these massive job losses but not in the less developed economies. This has resulted in significant long-term damage to many young families around the world.

Fiscal impact: Economies around the world experienced significant contractions, with negative GDP growth in many countries. The pandemic-induced recession rivaled the severity of the great depression in some regions. Lockdowns and reduced consumer spending led to decreased economic activity. Many businesses, particularly small and medium-sized enterprises (SMEs), were forced to close permanently due to revenue losses and the inability to cover fixed costs during lockdowns. The closure of businesses disrupted supply chains and resulted in lost livelihoods for entrepreneurs and employees. Global trade was severely disrupted due to restrictions on movement, border closures, and supply chain interruptions. Export-dependent economies faced challenges as demand for goods and services declined. Financial markets experienced extreme volatility, with stock markets witnessing rapid declines and recoveries. Investors grappled with uncertainty and market fluctuations.

Central banks implemented monetary policies to stabilize markets and support liquidity. Many governments also implemented stimulus packages and relief measures to cushion the economic impact. These measures included direct payments to individuals, financial support for businesses, and unemployment benefits. These interventions resulted in increased government debt levels and budget deficits. However, the economic impact of COVID-19 disproportionately affected vulnerable populations, exacerbating income and wealth inequalities. Low-income workers, minorities, and those in informal sectors faced greater challenges in accessing healthcare, financial support, and remote work opportunities. Economists have raised concerns about potential long-term economic scarring, including the erosion of human capital, diminished productivity, and lasting business closures. The pandemic may have lasting effects on the structure and dynamics of industries.

Digital transformation acceleration: In a silver lining to the dark cloud of COVID-19, it accelerated digital transformation, with businesses pivoting to e-commerce, remote work, and online services (LaBerge et al., 2020). Firms that adapted quickly to digital strategies fared better during the crisis (Hai et al., 2021). COVID-19 accelerated digital transformation in various ways, pushing organizations, governments, and individuals to adopt and rely on digital technologies more rapidly than they might have otherwise. For example, faced with lockdowns and social distancing measures, many organizations quickly transitioned to remote work, also called popularly as work-from-home (WFH). This led to the rapid adoption of communication and collaboration tools such as Zoom, Microsoft Teams, WebEx, and others. Similarly, as physical stores faced closures or reduced capacity, e-commerce surged in demand, with consumers increasingly shopping online for a wide range of goods, from groceries to electronics. Figure 2.3 shows the acceleration of digitization of customer interactions during COVID-19.

The pandemic also led to a surge in telehealth and virtual medical consultations as people preferred to seek medical advice and services remotely as far as possible in order to minimize exposure to the virus, and in response, healthcare providers rapidly adopted digital tools for consultations, prescriptions,

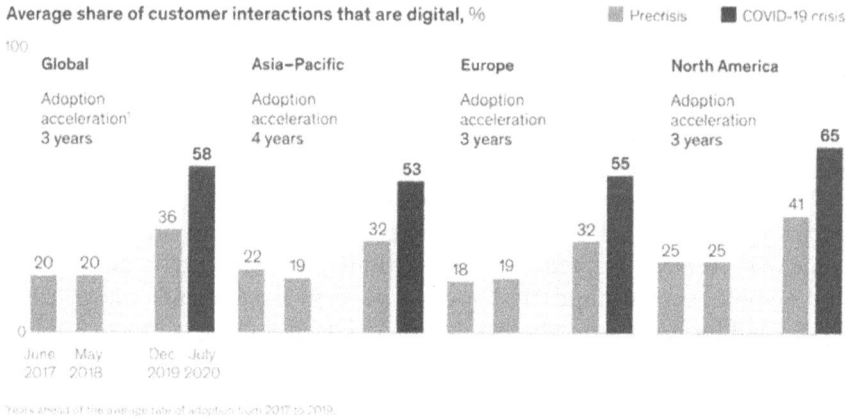

Average share of customer interactions that are digital, %   ▓ Precrisis   ■ COVID-19 crisis

Figure 2.3 Acceleration of digitization during COVID-19

and monitoring (Bhatt et al., 2020). With schools and universities closed for indefinite periods, educators and students also had to quickly adapt to online learning platforms and digital tools for remote education (Mittal et al., 2022). Another major outcome of the pandemic was the rapid adoption of digital payment systems (e.g., mobile wallets, contactless cards, and other online payment platforms) in response to concerns about the spread of the virus via physical currency, especially in the emerging markets like India (Jain et al., 2020). Other businesses, especially those in traditional industries such as financial services and higher education, expedited their migration to cloud-based infrastructure to support remote work, enhance scalability, and reduce reliance on physical hardware (Sharma et al., 2023).

Many businesses also strived to enhance the visibility and resilience of their supply chains by adopting digital tools for tracking and managing inventory, production, and logistics (Panwar et al., 2022). The pandemic also highlighted the need for data-driven decision-making and organizations increasingly turned to data analytics and artificial intelligence to gain insights, automate processes, and make informed choices (Agarwal et al., 2022). Similarly, with an increased reliance on digital tools, there was a heightened awareness of the importance of cybersecurity and data protection, which led to increased investment in security measures (Lallie et al., 2021). Interestingly, businesses such as meetings, events, conferences, and trade shows, which were adversely affected by COVID-19 with restrictions on travel and public gatherings due to social distancing measures, managed to survive by shifting to virtual formats (Jaafar & Khan, 2022). This in turn led to many innovations in virtual event platforms and technologies for hosting and attending large-scale gatherings online (Bukovska et al., 2021). Similarly, with theaters and live events being shut down, streaming services for movies, TV shows, and live performances experienced a surge in popularity (Ryu & Cho, 2022).

Finally, even governments around the world accelerated the digitization of public services to provide citizens with online access to essential services, such as healthcare information, unemployment benefits, and government assistance (Mansour, 2022). Hence, it can be seen clearly that COVID-19 has acted as a catalyst, driving organizations and individuals to innovate and adapt to a rapidly changing landscape. While these digital transformations were driven by necessity, many of the changes are likely to have a lasting impact on how businesses and society operate in the post-pandemic world. For example, most universities around the world have maintained the hybrid mode of teaching, retaining a combination of online lectures and in-person tutorials (Adedoyin & Soykan, 2023; Li, 2022). Similarly, healthcare service providers, especially those in the public sector and managed by governments, tried to use online platforms to maintain the continuity of their essential services as far as possible.

2.3 Education disruption

The pandemic disrupted education systems worldwide with school closures forcing students to transition to remote learning, exposing them to the challenges of providing quality education in online mode (Karalis, 2020). Many students faced difficulties accessing technology resulting in a digital divide, while others struggled with the absence of face-to-face interactions with teachers and peers. COVID-19 triggered a seismic disruption in the field of education, impacting students, teachers, parents, and educational institutions worldwide (García-Morales et al., 2021). The impact of disrupted education could have long-term consequences on learning outcomes and future opportunities (Mohd-Dom et al., 2022). This section outlines the profound effects and transformations caused by COVID-19 in the realm of education in schools, colleges, and universities around the world. Figure 2.4 shows learning delays during COVID-19, with the most severe impact in the countries with prolonged restrictions (Bryant et al., 2022).

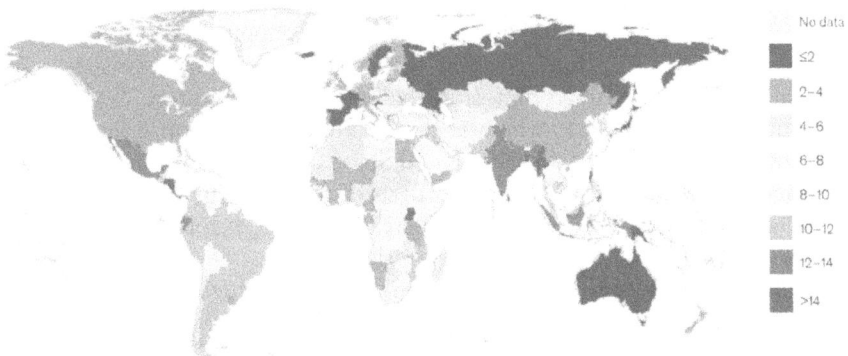

Figure 2.4 Estimated learning delays in months by country (February 2020–January 2022)

Source: https://www.mckinsey.com/industries/education/our-insights

School closures and shift to remote learning: One of the most immediate and visible impacts was the closure of schools and educational institutions in numerous countries. Lockdowns and social distancing measures necessitated the suspension of in-person classes to curb the spread of the virus (Viner et al., 2020). To continue education during lockdowns, a rapid shift to remote learning occurred. Schools, colleges, and universities adopted online platforms and digital tools to deliver lessons. This transition highlighted disparities in access to technology and internet connectivity, affecting students' ability to participate in remote learning. Remote learning poses challenges for students, teachers, and parents alike (Tulaskar & Turunen, 2022). Students faced difficulties in adapting to virtual classrooms, maintaining focus, and staying motivated. Teachers had to adapt their instructional methods and tools, learn new technologies and applications, and find new ways to engage students online. Parents also had to take on additional roles as educators at home to supplement their children's learning and faced the challenge of balancing work responsibilities with their children's education.

Educational inequalities and mental health impact: The pandemic exacerbated educational inequalities. Students from lower-income households often lacked access to necessary devices, a quiet study environment, and parental support (Haelermans et al., 2022). These disparities in access to education disproportionately affected marginalized and vulnerable populations. The disruption in traditional education took a toll on the mental health and well-being of students. Social isolation, disrupted routines, and uncertainty about the future contributed to increased stress and anxiety (Chaturvedi et al., 2021).

Innovation and digital transformation: Despite challenges, the pandemic accelerated innovation in education with educational technology (EdTech) companies, video conferencing platforms, and online learning platforms experiencing significant growth as educators worldwide embraced innovative teaching methods, including gamified learning, virtual field trips, and interactive online content. According to a recent report by the CFI Group, the global EdTech sector is expected to grow rapidly from $12.8 billion in 2020 to $81.2 billion by 2030, reflecting a compounded annual growth rate (CAGR) of 20.5%, triggered by technological developments and changes in the education sector (Schuitevoerder, 2023). Hence, it is not surprising to see the EdTech market attracts almost 21 billion dollars of venture capital (VC) funding globally in 2021, which is three times the 7 billion dollars in VC funding it attracted in 2019. The United States accounts for most of these investments although Europe and other parts of the world are also catching up. Thus, online education is playing an increasingly bigger role, especially since COVID-19, offering new data for new insights.

Hybrid and blended learning models: Some educational institutions adopted hybrid or blended learning models, combining in-person and online instruction, to mitigate the effects of school closures. These models offered flexibility while adhering to health guidelines. Traditional methods of assessment and evaluation faced limitations in the remote learning environment.

Educators had to adapt assessments to measure student learning effectively, which in turn raised questions about the fairness and validity of remote testing. However, it is clear that many of these changes may continue during the post-pandemic era due to their positive impact on the efficiency of teaching delivery and engagement (Al-Hunaiyyan et al., 2021).

Future of education: The pandemic prompted discussions about the future of education. Many educators and institutions are re-evaluating the role of technology, remote learning, and the classroom experience in post-pandemic education. COVID-19 has reshaped the landscape of education and prompted a reimagining of traditional teaching methods and learning environments. With all the ongoing changes, the professional development of educators has become quite critical to enhance their digital skills, adapt to new teaching modalities, and ensure effective remote instruction. While the challenges have been substantial, the crisis has also spurred innovation, collaboration, and a broader recognition of the importance of adaptable, resilient education systems that can navigate unforeseen disruptions.

2.4 Mental health challenges

The pandemic has exacerbated mental health issues globally. Isolation, uncertainty, fear, and grief take a toll on individuals' mental well-being. Lockdowns and social distancing measures limited social interactions and support networks, contributing to feelings of loneliness and anxiety. Frontline healthcare workers and vulnerable populations faced particularly high levels of stress. The mental health crisis highlighted the need for increased mental health resources and support. COVID-19 has not only unleashed a global health crisis but has also cast a stark light on the mental health challenges faced by individuals and communities around the world. The invisible toll of the pandemic on mental well-being has been profound and multifaceted. This description outlines the mental health challenges posed by COVID-19. Figure 2.5 shows an uneven impact of COVID-19 on global mental health, as indicated by the sharp increase in the number of mental disorders during the pandemic across 204 countries and territories around the world, particularly among younger people and females (Santomauro et al., 2021).

Isolation and loneliness: Loneliness and social isolation generally co-exist and are more common in older adults compared to other age groups because they are more likely to be out of work, suffer from poor health, and live away from their family members. However, these are not the same, as loneliness refers to people's subjective feelings, whereas social isolation is the level and frequency of one's social interactions. More specifically, loneliness is defined as the subjective feeling of being alone, while social isolation is defined as an objective state of social environment and interaction patterns. Thus, although loneliness and social isolation are not equal to each other, both can have a devastating impact on people's mental health through a combination of many common as well as independent mechanisms, which became activated by the

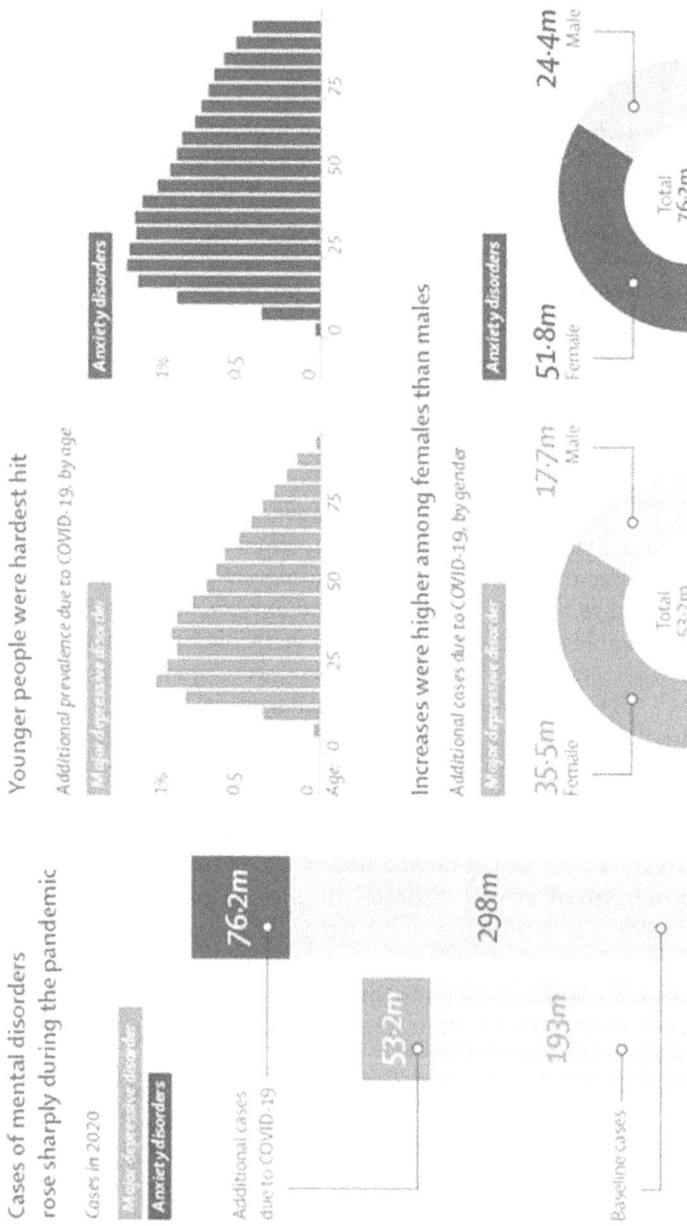

Figure 2.5 Uneven impact of COVID-19 on global mental health (Yoch & Sirull, 2021)

Source: *https://www.healthdata.org/news-events/insights-blog*

pandemic (Hwang et al., 2020). For example, frequent and extended lock-downs, strict social distancing measures, and prolonged quarantine protocols resulted in widespread isolation and loneliness, with many individuals being separated from loved ones, leading to feelings of loneliness and disconnection. These symptoms were particularly severe among the older people as many of them were locked out and could not meet their loved ones due to fears about their health and well-being (Williams et al., 2021).

Anxiety and fear: The uncertainty and fear surrounding the virus triggered heightened levels of anxiety due to concerns about personal health, the health of loved ones, and economic stability have been sources of significant stress (Coelho et al., 2020). COVID-19 presented a very serious multifaceted global mental health challenge affecting almost every aspect of human life and disrupting the social fabric in the process. It triggered several fears among the population, ranging from contamination, financial instability, and insecurity about the future to even extreme reactions like agoraphobia and xenophobia. This situation presented significant challenges for physicians, other healthcare workers, and first responders such as police officers, fire-fighters, and rescue personnel, as they were not trained to deal with people and situations involving these fears and anxiety related to COVID-19 (Coelho et al., 2020).

Grief and loss: The pandemic has brought loss and grief to the forefront. Many have lost family members, friends, or colleagues to COVID-19, and the inability to hold traditional funerals and memorial services has complicated the grieving process (Kumar, 2023). A unique feature of the grief and loss experienced during COVID-19 was that people may not have had enough time to completely get over the painful effects due to the prolonged nature of the pandemic. Another important aspect of the individual experiences particularly relevant to the pandemic was that they experienced multiple losses, including loss of loved ones, employment and livelihood, identity, poor health outcomes, and significant life events. A failure to address the needs of those people who experienced loss and grief during COVID-19 may result in poor long-term mental and physical health for them. Hence, it is important to recognize and acknowledge the uniqueness of each individual's experience of their loss and grief to guide mental health experts and service providers to develop customized actions to help them cope with their loss and promote their mental health and overall well-being (Zhai & Du, 2020).

Uncertainty about the future: The uncertainty surrounding the duration and impact of the pandemic created a sense of powerlessness and hopelessness for many people as their personal and professional plans and aspirations were put on hold or disrupted (Stuart et al., 2021). Economic instability resulting from job losses, furloughs, and business closures also contributed to financial stress for many people, which in turn affected their mental health, as they struggled to meet their basic needs, including food, clothing, housing, and transportation. COVID-19 also led to a substantial increase in the financial uncertainty as reflected by lower returns on stocks listed in both, S&P 500 and Nasdaq Composite index (Shehzad et al., 2020)

Disruption of daily routine and work-life: The disruption of daily routines, including work, school, and social activities, during COVID-19 left many people feeling directionless and struggling to find a sense of structure and purpose (Sangster Jokić & Jokić-Begić, 2022). Essential workers, healthcare professionals, and educators, in particular, faced overwhelming workloads, often without adequate support, which led to burnout and mental exhaustion (Hite & McDonald, 2020). With the shift to remote work, many employees transitioned to working from home to comply with social distancing measures, which required adjustments to home setups and the adoption of new work schedules and tools. Shifts to online learning disrupted traditional education systems, presenting challenges for students, parents, and educators. With the closure of schools and childcare centers, parents had to juggle work responsibilities with childcare and homeschooling duties. With most offices closed, people stayed home and did not have to commute, which affected public transportation systems, traffic patterns, and related industries. The closure of theaters, restaurants, bars, and other entertainment venues limited recreational options for individuals and families. Access to gyms, recreational facilities, and wellness services was restricted, leading to changes in exercise and self-care routines.

Social distancing measures led to reduced face-to-face interactions as people could not go out for shopping or recreation, which also impacted their mental health and social well-being. Isolation, uncertainty, and anxiety induced by all the movement restrictions and lockdowns due to the pandemic had a significant impact on mental health of many individuals. Many individuals faced job losses, furloughs, or financial instability, leading to concerns about economic well-being. Restrictions on operations and reduced consumer spending led to closures and financial challenges for many small businesses and sectors like hospitality and tourism. Travel restrictions, reduced flights, and concerns about virus transmission affected travel plans and the tourism industry. Even routine healthcare services, elective procedures, and non-COVID-19-related treatments were often delayed or modified due to the strain on healthcare systems. The need for increased hygiene measures, mask-wearing, and social distancing became integral parts of daily routines. People became more conscious of health practices, including hand hygiene, respiratory etiquette, and vaccination. Overall, most families struggled to cope with the challenges and stress posed by the pandemic (Bates et al., 2021).

Impact on vulnerable populations: Vulnerable populations, including those with pre-existing mental health issues, substance use disorders, and limited access to healthcare, were disproportionately affected by the mental health impacts of the pandemic (Silliman Cohen & Bosk, 2020). For example, vulnerable populations, such as the elderly, those with underlying health conditions, and those living in congregate settings like nursing homes, experienced higher infection and mortality rates. Similarly, minority communities, such as Black, Indigenous, and Latino populations in the US, were disproportionately affected, with higher infection rates, hospitalizations, and deaths due to systemic inequalities in healthcare access and socio-economic factors. Vulnerable populations face challenges in accessing healthcare services, including testing, treatment, and preventive care due to a lack of adequate insurance. Homeless individuals and those in crowded, inadequate housing faced higher risks of infection due to difficulties in maintaining social distancing and practicing good hygiene. Others, including those with pre-existing mental health conditions or experiencing economic hardship, faced heightened stress, anxiety, depression, and other mental health challenges.

Low-income individuals and families, as well as those working in gig economy jobs or in sectors heavily impacted by the pandemic (e.g., hospitality, retail, service industries), experienced job loss, income instability, and financial strain. Many vulnerable populations, including essential workers, faced higher risks of exposure due to the nature of their jobs. This included healthcare workers, grocery store employees, transportation workers, and others. Closure of schools, disruption of social activities, and uncertainty about the future took a toll on the mental health of children and adolescents, with a dramatic increase in anxiety and depression among young people (Masonbrink & Hurley, 2020). Children from lower-income families in particular, often lacked the resources and technology for effective online learning, and therefore, school closures disproportionately affected their education. Older adults, especially those living in long-term care facilities, also experienced significant isolation due to restrictions on visitation, leading to mental health challenges. Initial disparities in vaccine distribution and access further highlighted existing inequalities, as vulnerable populations faced challenges in securing timely vaccinations.

People without access to reliable internet or digital devices faced challenges in accessing critical information, telehealth services, and remote work or education opportunities. Vulnerable populations, including low-income families and individuals, and even foreign students with no insurance coverage for COVID-19 and loss of their part-time jobs, faced increased food insecurity due to disruptions in the food supply chain and economic instability (Gundersen et al., 2021). Those in congregate settings such as correctional facilities, homeless shelters, and migrant worker housing faced higher risks of outbreaks due to close living quarters and challenges in implementing preventive measures. Language barriers, limited health literacy, and lack of access to reliable information posed challenges in understanding and following public health guidelines (Sauer et al., 2021). All these adverse impacts underscored the urgent need for targeted interventions, equity-focused policies, and support systems to address the unique challenges faced by vulnerable populations during the pandemic.

Access to mental health services: Many individuals have faced barriers to accessing mental health services due to overwhelmed healthcare systems, reduced availability of in-person services, and stigma associated with seeking help (Egede et al., 2020; Saltzman et al., 2021). The increased reliance on digital communication for work, education, and social interaction has led to "Zoom fatigue" and screen time-related mental health challenges, although these innovations are now being seen as almost inevitable in the post-COVID-19 era (Bullock et al., 2022). According to some researchers, the severe mental health challenges posed by COVID-19 were like a silent pandemic within the larger crisis as these transcend geographic boundaries, affecting people of all ages, backgrounds, and circumstances (Tsamakis et al., 2021). The importance of addressing mental health alongside physical health during and after the pandemic cannot be overstated. Initiatives to promote mental well-being, reduce stigma, and expand access to mental health services are essential components of a comprehensive response to COVID-19. Despite the challenges, many individuals have demonstrated remarkable resilience and adaptability, through coping strategies such as mindfulness, exercise, and connecting with loved ones through virtual means (Backhaus et al., 2021).

2.5   Inequality amplification

COVID-19 disproportionately affected vulnerable and marginalized populations, amplifying existing inequalities with low-income workers, informal sector laborers, and marginalized communities facing much greater economic and health risks compared to others (Patel et al., 2020a). Women, who often bear the brunt of caregiving responsibilities, were disproportionately affected as they grappled with increased domestic burdens and job losses (Fortier, 2020). COVID-19 has acted as a magnifying glass, exposing and exacerbating pre-existing inequalities in societies around the world, with a combination of factors leaving the most economically disadvantaged people particularly vulnerable to COVID-19. These factors include greater exposure to the virus, pre-existing comorbidities and stress associated with poverty, and poorer access to healthcare for the disadvantaged sections of the society. The pandemic not only revealed the stark inequalities within society but also made them worse (Patel et al., 2020a). To address the vulnerabilities of the most economically disadvantaged group within society, policymakers must introduce long-term legislation to improve social welfare (Mishra et al., 2021). This section explores the ways in which the pandemic has amplified socioeconomic disparities, leaving vulnerable populations even more marginalized.

Economic disparities: The pandemic's economic impact has disproportionately affected low-income individuals and communities, with greater job losses, business closures, and reduced work hours, leading to financial instability, particularly for those in precarious employment. In fact, economic disparity and inequality may have even led to excess mortality rates during COVID-19 (Zaki et al., 2022), through unfair labor market structures (resulting in disproportionate representation in industrial and other high-risk jobs) and income inequalities (representing asymmetry and concentration at the lower end of income distributions). The amplification of socioeconomic disparities during COVID-19 highlights the urgent need for equitable and inclusive policies and interventions. Addressing these inequalities requires targeted efforts to ensure that vulnerable populations have access to healthcare, education, economic support, and vaccination. The pandemic has underscored the interconnectedness of our world and the imperative of building more resilient and equitable societies for the future.

Access to healthcare: Vulnerable populations, including those without adequate health insurance or access to healthcare facilities, faced challenges in seeking COVID-19 testing, treatment, and vaccination, with racial and ethnic minorities often experiencing disparities in healthcare access and outcomes in particular (Clay et al., 2021). Racial and ethnic minorities, along with low-income individuals, experienced higher rates of COVID-19 infections, hospitalizations, and deaths. Underlying health disparities contributed to these outcomes. Access to COVID-19 vaccines has been unequal, with wealthier countries securing a majority of the early vaccine supplies. This has left poorer nations with limited access to vaccines, prolonging the global pandemic. For example, more non-Hispanic Blacks (61.1%) and Whites (61.2%) experienced a higher severity risk of COVID-19 compared to Hispanics (47.1%). In addition, these racial differences were accentuated for females, unmarried, unemployed, limited access to transportation, and poor affordability to pay for medicines. Being non-Hispanic Black and older, having appointment issues and affordability issues with medicine were also associated with increased severity risk of COVID-19 (Clay et al., 2021). All these findings have important implications for the design and planning of public healthcare facilities in future to minimize these disparities and their catastrophic outcomes. Figure 2.6 highlights the different types of inequalities triggered by the COVID-19 pandemic according to Oxfam (2021).

Remote work disparities: The ability to work remotely became a privilege during the pandemic, allowing some to maintain their income and job security (Daneshfar et al., 2023). However, this option was not available to many frontline workers especially in service industries, resulting in disparities in job security. Essential workers, who are often from marginalized communities, also face higher risks of exposure to the virus due to the nature of their jobs and because they often lack the option to work from home or adequate protective equipment and measures in place. Notwithstanding this, most people felt positive in general about being able to work remotely during the pandemic as it allowed them to balance their work and home lives, although they also faced a few challenges, including limited space and time to work freely at home, lack of recreational activities and support mechanisms, and having to balance household chores and carer duties while working at the same time. Moreover, many people reported feeling exhausted and stressed out in trying to balance their work with home responsibilities, and the fear of losing their jobs and coping strategies to deal with the uncertainty seemed to help them overcome these challenges.

Education disparities: School closures and the shift to remote learning exposed disparities in access to technology, internet connectivity, and a conducive learning environment, wherein the students from low-income households

THE INEQUALITY VIRUS

It took just NINE MONTHS for the fortunes of the top 1,000 billionaires to return to their pre-pandemic highs, while for the world's poorest, recovery could take MORE THAN A DECADE.

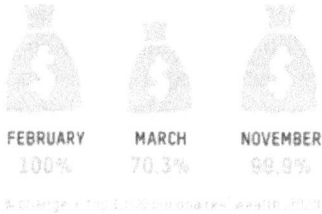

THE INCREASE in the wealth of the 10 richest billionaires since the crisis began IS MORE THAN ENOUGH to prevent anyone on Earth from falling into poverty because of the virus and to pay for a COVID-19 vaccine for all.

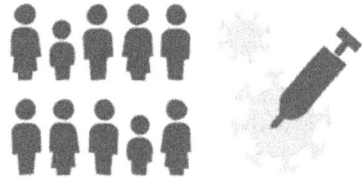

FEBRUARY	MARCH	NOVEMBER
100%	70.3%	98.9%

% change in top 1,000 billionaires' wealth, 2020

In the US, CLOSE TO 22,000 LATINX AND BLACK PEOPLE would have still been alive as of December 2020 if these communities' COVID-19 mortality rates were the same as WHITE PEOPLE'S.

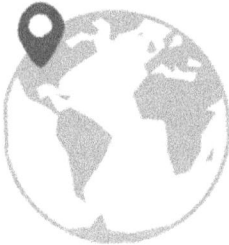

112 MILLION FEWER WOMEN would be at high risk of losing their incomes or jobs if women and men were equally represented in sectors negatively affected by the COVID-19 crisis.

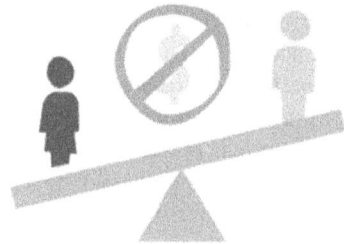

Oxfam's survey of economists on the impact of the coronavirus pandemic on inequality found that:

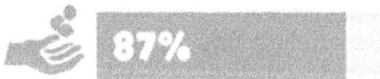

87% of respondents think that coronavirus will lead to an increase or a major increase in INCOME INEQUALITY in their country.

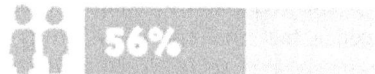

56% of respondents think that coronavirus will likely or very likely lead to an increase in GENDER INEQUALITY in their country.

Figure 2.6 The inequality virus (Oxfam, 2021)
Source: Oxfam (https://oxfamilibrary.openrepository.com)

often lacked the resources to participate fully in online education (Mason-brink & Hurley, 2020). Educational disparities become quite visible as the switch to remote learning methods and e-learning as a mode of instruction experienced inequitable access for students from disadvantaged backgrounds (Allen et al., 2022). As students from racial and ethnic minorities, often live in communities with significant social, economic, and educational disparities; they did not have access to multiple devices – good quality broadband internet and parents who could supplement their learning by working from home. As a result, indiscriminate adoption of e-learning may have contributed to and reinforced inequitable education policies as it failed to acknowledge significant disadvantages experienced by students from racial and ethnic minority backgrounds (Allen et al., 2022). In addition, vulnerable children and adolescents, including those in foster care or without stable homes, experienced significant disruptions in education and lacked the support structures available to many others, such as laptops, tablets, and a good quality internet connection.

Mental health inequalities: Vulnerable populations, including individuals with pre-existing mental health conditions, experienced disparities in access to mental health services due to all the restrictions imposed during the pandemic, and this in turn further compounded the pandemic's impact on the mental health and well-being of those with limited access to support (Gibson et al., 2021). In particular, researchers found significantly higher mental health inequalities for females, young people, financially insecure, with lack of access to clear information about the pandemic, proximity to large infection sites, existing physical/psychological health conditions, and being subjected to abuse or stigma because of their identity as a member of an ethnic or sexual marginalized group (Gibson et al., 2021).

Housing insecurity: The economic fallout from the pandemic led to housing insecurity and homelessness for many individuals and families as those living in overcrowded or substandard housing faced higher risks of COVID-19 transmission. In addition, many landlords forced their tenants to pay much higher rents or vacate their houses on flimsy pretexts, which further aggravated the housing situation for the most vulnerable sections of the society (Versey, 2021). As the coronavirus rampaged through the United States, more than 40 million people lost their jobs and faced challenges in paying their rents, mortgages, property taxes, and utilities (Mehdipanah, 2020). Although subsequent moratoria on evictions and foreclosures coupled with deferral of mortgage payments helped people avoid becoming homeless during the pandemic, these programs could not provide long-term protection to those who lost income or faced financial uncertainty due to either their own poor health and long-term consequences of catching the virus or the loss of their loved ones, in particular the working members in the family. Thus, it is estimated that the increasing financial insecurity and the chronic shortage of affordable housing will continue to affect the lower-income households even in the aftermath of COVID-19. For these households, any prolonged financial hardships will lead to millions of them risk losing their homes through evictions and foreclosures.

Gender disparities: The pandemic disproportionately affected women, who often shouldered increased caregiving responsibilities and faced job losses in sectors heavily impacted by the crisis, such as hospitality and retail (Singh et al., 2022; Villarreal & Yu, 2022). As governments around the world reacted with swift and strict measures to control the pandemic's spread, these actions may have disproportionately increased the risks for women, both directly and indirectly (Gausman & Langer, 2020). For example, pregnant women are among the most vulnerable groups during public health emergencies as they are more biologically susceptible to adverse health outcomes, such as respiratory infections. Similarly, pregnant women are more likely than non-pregnant women to experience severe complications if they are infected by the COVID-19 virus. In addition, women are generally more likely to perform the role of a carer and also take care of the everyday chores in most households around the world, which put them under extra mental stress and physical strain due to the unique challenges posed by COVID-19, such as all family members including children, adults, and the elderly, spending more time at home. In fact, there is significant evidence of the rise of domestic violence towards women during the pandemic (Kourti et al., 2023)

2.6   Balancing global competition and cooperation

The pandemic strained global cooperation and highlighted the shortcomings of international institutions. Nationalistic responses and a lack of coordinated efforts hindered the global response to the crisis. Vaccine distribution disparities showcased inequities in access to life-saving resources. The pandemic underscored the need for stronger international collaboration to address global challenges effectively, as seen in the global concerted efforts to develop effective vaccines and other remedies. COVID-19, while a global threat, has also revealed and intensified existing strains on international cooperation. This description outlines the ways in which the pandemic has tested unity among nations and international organizations.

Vaccine nationalism: The pursuit of COVID-19 vaccines and critical medical supplies by wealthy nations, termed "vaccine nationalism" came at the expense of equitable global distribution, which hindered global efforts to ensure that all nations had equitable access to vaccines (Hassoun, 2021). Vaccine nationalism is defined as the prioritization of domestic needs of a country for vaccine dosages while ignoring the needs of other countries with the aim of improving their own protection and reducing vulnerability against the virus. However, vaccinating people in their own country and ignoring others may be a foolproof safeguard as the virus would still be out there and could return to one's own country anytime in the future. In other words, the virus would continue to mutate in other countries and may eventually erode the immune response set out by the old vaccines, which would nullify all the efforts made in the development, production, distribution, and administration of the vaccines (Lagman, 2021).

Vaccine diplomacy: Some nations engaged in "vaccine diplomacy", using vaccine distribution as a tool for advancing their geopolitical interests, which introduced competition rather than collaboration (Sparke & Levy, 2022). For example, India emerged as the vaccine manufacturing hub of the world, contributing 60% to the global vaccine supply with the capacity to manufacture well over three billion COVID-19 vaccine doses annually (Sharun & Dhama, 2021). Hence, India was able to leverage its unique position to produce low-cost COVID-19 vaccines and share those with low-income countries that either could not afford or were not allowed to buy the expensive vaccines manufactured by the developed countries (Sharun & Dhama, 2021). In fact, India also supplied its vaccines to the more developed countries like Australia, the Netherlands, and UK, resulting in a total export of more than 300 million doses by June 2023. By contrast, China tried to use its vaccines not only to repair its image in the aftermath of COVID-19 outbreak in Wuhan and to continue its ambitions for greater global expansion of its power, but to also reinforce and leverage its existing soft power initiatives by capitalizing on new economic and geopolitical opportunities (Lee, 2023). Sentiment analyses of social media and international media coverage indicate an improvement in China's image and influence with its vaccine diplomacy but significant concerns over Chinese vaccines' efficacy, safety, and data availability still remain, especially among its rival global powers.

Export restrictions: Some countries imposed export restrictions on medical supplies, including personal protective equipment (PPE) and ventilators, limiting the ability of other nations to access essential equipment during the crisis (Hoekman et al., 2020). These policies break supply chains that rely on sourcing inputs from different countries, reduce access to critically needed supplies and foster excessive price spikes and volatility, and generate foreign policy tensions. Experience with widespread use of export restrictions by food exporting countries in times of market disruption and supply shortages suggests a priority for the G20 should be to work with industry to put in place systems to enhance access to information on production capacity, investments to boost supplies and address supply chain bottlenecks affecting production and trade in essential medical supplies (Espitia et al., 2020).

Travel restrictions: During the early stages of the pandemic, unilateral travel bans and restrictions were implemented by many countries, often without coordination or consultation with other countries, resulting in unprecedented shutdown of borders and airlines, which in turn disrupted global travel and trade, and severely restricted the free movement of essential medical supplies and healthcare workers that were vital to control the spread of the virus and to save lives (Devi, 2020). Others find that the travel ban out of Wuhan delayed the overall epidemic progression by only 3 to 5 days in mainland China but it did slow down the spread outside China by about 80% until mid-February 2020, although it was difficult to control the spread within each country due to limited impact of local restrictions (Chinazzi et al., 2020).

Disinformation and miscommunication: The spread of misinformation and disinformation regarding COVID-19 complicated international cooperation efforts as false narratives and conspiracy theories hindered trust and information sharing (Gottlieb & Dyer, 2020). The sharing of critical scientific and epidemiological data also faced many hurdles, including issues related to data sovereignty and concerns about the misuse of sensitive information.

The pandemic also saw a dramatic rise in medical disinformation on social media with a wide variety of claims, including COVID-19 vaccine being a hoax or deliberately manufactured in a lab by some countries, 5G frequency radiation causing the illness, and being a trick by big pharmaceutical companies to make profits from a vaccine later (Grimes, 2021). These findings present a unique challenge to the governments and health authorities around the world to prepare themselves to counter such disinformation campaigns in future. Figure 2.7 shows the nine key themes of COVID-19 disinfodemic (UNESCO, 2020).

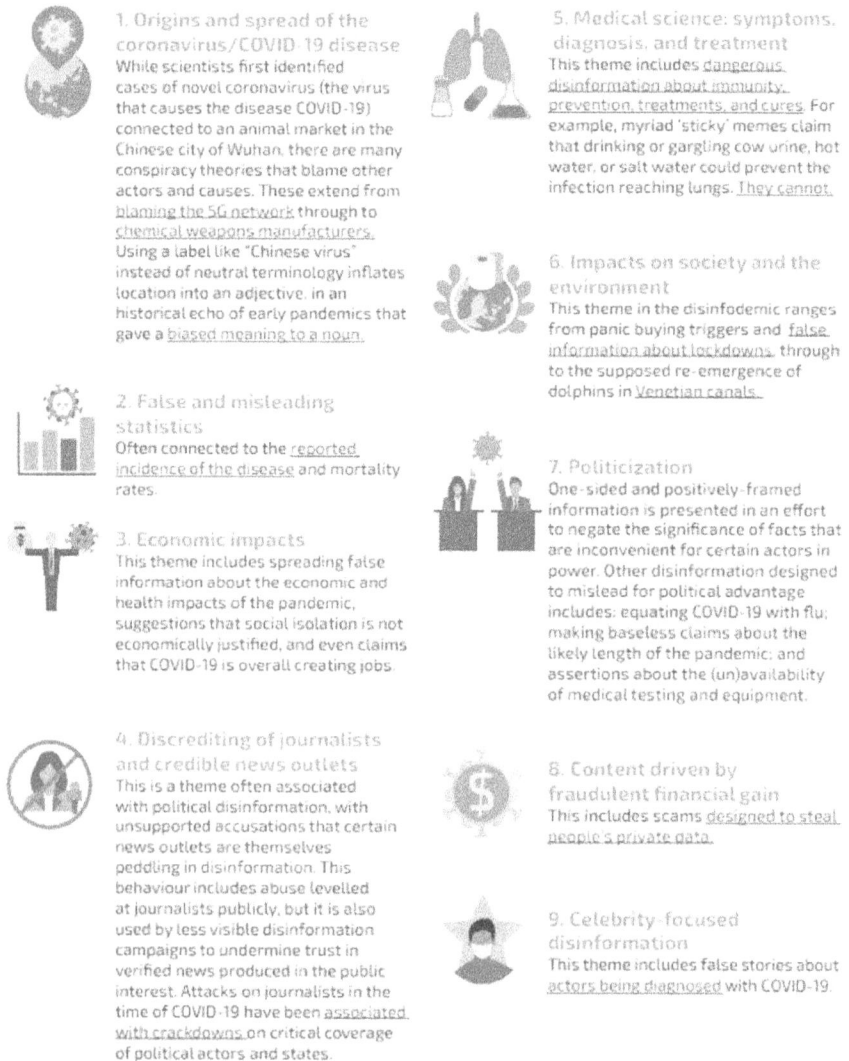

1. Origins and spread of the coronavirus/COVID-19 disease
While scientists first identified cases of novel coronavirus (the virus that causes the disease COVID-19) connected to an animal market in the Chinese city of Wuhan, there are many conspiracy theories that blame other actors and causes. These extend from blaming the 5G network through to chemical weapons manufacturers. Using a label like "Chinese virus" instead of neutral terminology inflates location into an adjective, in an historical echo of early pandemics that gave a biased meaning to a noun.

2. False and misleading statistics
Often connected to the reported incidence of the disease and mortality rates.

3. Economic impacts
This theme includes spreading false information about the economic and health impacts of the pandemic, suggestions that social isolation is not economically justified, and even claims that COVID-19 is overall creating jobs.

4. Discrediting of journalists and credible news outlets
This is a theme often associated with political disinformation, with unsupported accusations that certain news outlets are themselves peddling in disinformation. This behaviour includes abuse levelled at journalists publicly, but it is also used by less visible disinformation campaigns to undermine trust in verified news produced in the public interest. Attacks on journalists in the time of COVID-19 have been associated with crackdowns on critical coverage of political actors and states.

5. Medical science: symptoms, diagnosis, and treatment
This theme includes dangerous disinformation about immunity, prevention, treatments, and cures. For example, myriad 'sticky' memes claim that drinking or gargling cow urine, hot water, or salt water could prevent the infection reaching lungs. They cannot.

6. Impacts on society and the environment
This theme in the disinfodemic ranges from panic buying triggers and false information about lockdowns, through to the supposed re-emergence of dolphins in Venetian canals.

7. Politicization
One-sided and positively-framed information is presented in an effort to negate the significance of facts that are inconvenient for certain actors in power. Other disinformation designed to mislead for political advantage includes: equating COVID-19 with flu; making baseless claims about the likely length of the pandemic; and assertions about the (un)availability of medical testing and equipment.

8. Content driven by fraudulent financial gain
This includes scams designed to steal people's private data.

9. Celebrity-focused disinformation
This theme includes false stories about actors being diagnosed with COVID-19.

Figure 2.7 Nine key themes of COVID-19 disinfodemic (UNESCO, 2020)

Source: UNESCO (https://unesdoc.unesco.org)

Uneven distribution of resources: Global efforts to provide financial support to nations in need, particularly in the Global South, faced obstacles due to competing domestic priorities and economic challenges in donor countries (Rydland et al., 2022). Many low-income countries struggled to access COVID-19 testing and treatments due to supply chain disruptions and financial constraints, despite international efforts to provide assistance (Spieske & Birkel, 2021). Nations and organizations competed for limited supplies of medical equipment and vaccines, as the World Health Organization (WHO) and the United Nations (UN), faced challenges in coordinating a global response (Jana & Roy, 2021). Funding disputes, political tensions, and differing priorities strained their effectiveness (Lee & Haupt, 2021). Regional blocs and alliances also pursued their own responses to the pandemic, leading to fragmentation and competition rather than a coordinated global approach (Forman et al., 2020).

Delayed global response: While COVID-19 highlighted the importance of international cooperation, it also exposed fractures in the global system. The global response to the pandemic was often delayed, with nations initially adopting individualistic approaches before realizing the need for collaborative efforts (Filetti, 2020). Overcoming these strains and fostering greater unity in future crises will require concerted efforts to prioritize equity, share resources, and strengthen multilateral organizations (Cheng et al., 2022). The pandemic underscored the interconnectedness of our world and the imperative of collective action in the face of global threats. To summarize, the negative impact of COVID-19 has been far-reaching and multifaceted, touching upon every aspect of human life and society (Warne et al., 2020). COVID-19 exposed vulnerabilities, tested resilience, and highlighted the need for proactive measures to mitigate future crises. As the world moves forward, the lessons learned from this crisis can inform strategies to build more resilient, equitable, and prepared societies that can better withstand and respond to such challenges in the future (Kringos et al., 2020).

2.7   Conclusion

COVID-19's rapid global spread and the diverse reactions it elicited underscored humanity's shared vulnerability and resilience. The pandemic transcended borders, languages, and cultures, highlighting the interconnectedness of our world. The crisis prompted nations to reflect on their response strategies, laying the groundwork for more resilient and collaborative approaches to future challenges. As the world continues to grapple with the pandemic's aftermath, the lessons learned from its global spread and reactions will shape the trajectory of global health, governance, and solidarity. COVID-19 has highlighted the interdependence of global economies. International cooperation in areas like vaccine distribution, trade, and travel will be important for a coordinated and sustained economic recovery. Central banks have implemented various monetary measures to support economies during the pandemic.

Balancing inflation concerns with the need for continued economic stimulus will be a challenge. Ongoing geopolitical tensions (e.g., wars between Russia and Ukraine, Israel, and Hamas), trade disputes (e.g., China with Australia,

India, Japan, United States, and others), and other political factors can add additional layers of uncertainty to the economic recovery process (Sharif et al., 2020). The lessons learned from the pandemic may lead to increased investments in healthcare infrastructure, research, and preparedness, which could have long-term economic implications (Sharma et al., 2021). The pandemic has accelerated digital transformation, remote work, and other industry shifts, which may have long-term implications for the structure of economies and labor markets (Hai et al., 2021). Given the complexity and interdependence of these factors, predicting the exact trajectory of economic recovery remains challenging (Jaafar & Khan, 2022). A multidimensional approach, involving coordinated efforts from governments, businesses, and international organizations, will be crucial in navigating the uncertainties and fostering a resilient and sustainable recovery (Sharma et al., 2021).

As the virus's global footprint expanded, nations reacted in diverse ways to combat its spread. Responses ranged from swift, comprehensive lockdowns to more gradual containment measures. Countries like New Zealand adopted stringent measures early on, leading to effective virus suppression. In contrast, other nations struggled to balance health concerns with economic imperatives. The rapid spread of COVID-19 strained healthcare systems worldwide. Hospitals faced overwhelming patient loads, resulting in shortages of beds, ventilators, and medical personnel. These challenges prompted innovative solutions, such as repurposing facilities for COVID-19 care and rapid development of makeshift medical units. The pandemic's repercussions extended beyond health, profoundly impacting economies and societies. Lockdowns and travel restrictions led to job losses, business closures, and economic contraction. Vulnerable populations were disproportionately affected, highlighting the inequalities inherent in many societies.

COVID-19 catalyzed international collaboration in healthcare and research. Scientists across borders shared data, genetic information, and findings, expediting the development of diagnostic tests, treatments, and vaccines. Organizations like the WHO played a crucial role in coordinating efforts and disseminating guidelines. Communities rallied in the face of adversity. Acts of solidarity, such as mutual aid groups, volunteer efforts, and grassroots initiatives, demonstrated the resilience and empathy of individuals during times of crisis. People adapted to new norms, embracing remote work, virtual gatherings, and innovative methods of communication. However, the digital age brought with it the challenge of managing misinformation and an "infodemic". False claims, conspiracy theories, and misleading information proliferated, undermining public health efforts and sowing confusion. Combating this infodemic became a critical aspect of the global response.

2.8 Future lessons for managers

The rapid global spread of COVID-19 and its devastating socio-economic impact revealed the need for improved pandemic preparedness, international cooperation, and investment in healthcare infrastructure. It emphasized the importance of science-based decision-making and effective communication to build public trust. The crisis underscored the necessity of addressing social and economic disparities, as vulnerable communities were disproportionately affected. Economic disruption caused by COVID-19 is unprecedented in human history, with far-reaching consequences for individuals, businesses, and governments (Wang et al., 2023). The pandemic has emphasized the need for resilience, adaptability, and innovative solutions in the face of unforeseen challenges. Recovery efforts, fiscal policies, and global collaboration will play pivotal roles in shaping the post-pandemic economic landscape. The path to economic recovery remains uncertain, with the pace and shape of recovery varying by region and industry. Challenges such as vaccine distribution, new variants, and changing consumer behavior continue to impact recovery efforts. COVID-19 has introduced a high degree of uncertainty into the global economy, and its recovery trajectory remains uncertain.

First, the pace and success of vaccine distribution and administration played a crucial role in economic recovery, while at the same time, the emergence of new COVID-19 variants added an additional element of uncertainty, as it may have impacted the effectiveness of existing vaccines (Jacobs et al., 2023). Second, government policies and stimulus packages have been instrumental in stabilizing economies during the pandemic. However, the timing, size, and effectiveness of any similar future stimulus measures will be critical in determining the speed and sustainability of recovery (Stiglitz, 2021). Global supply chains were severely disrupted by the pandemic, affecting industries ranging from manufacturing to retail (Spieske & Birkel, 2021). Although food and other essential supplies were largely maintained throughout the pandemic, building more resilient supply chains would be a major priority to avoid any further disruptions to ensure a robust economic recovery. This could be achieved using emerging digital technologies, such as artificial intelligence and blockchain (Ozdemir et al., 2022).

The pandemic led to widespread job losses and disruptions in labor markets. The pace at which people return to the workforce and the extent to which industries have been able to rehire have also influenced economic recovery (Chang et al., 2022). For example, we can already see serious implications for small businesses such as restaurants, hair salons, boutiques, and other services, which are struggling to reopen and remain profitable, especially as many of them had to shut down during COVID-19 due to demand destruction and loss of key workers. Consumer confidence and behavior were significantly impacted by the pandemic but the growing willingness of consumers to spend, travel, and engage in activities that were restricted during lockdowns is playing a crucial role in economic recovery. Most small businesses faced serious challenges during the pandemic and their ability to survive, adapt, and grow in the post-pandemic landscape will have implications for overall economic recovery (Katare et al., 2021). The pandemic's economic impact may have long-lasting effects, particularly on certain sectors like travel, hospitality, and entertainment. Addressing these scars and supporting affected industries will be important for recovery (Rahman et al., 2021).

The COVID-19 pandemic disrupted global labor markets during 2020 and its short-term impact was very sudden and quite severe, with millions of people losing their jobs are being put on furlough (leave without pay), while others had to adjust very quickly to significant changes in their working conditions, such as work from home as many offices shut down due to the lockdowns and social distancing measures. Many workers were considered essential, such as bus and truck drivers, delivery persons, hospital and grocery store employees, garbage movers and warehouse workers, and they had to continue working albeit under new protocols to reduce the spread of the virus. A recent report by McKinsey on the future of work argues that many of these changes introduced during COVID-19 may remain even after the pandemic is gone (Lund et al., 2021). For example, remote work and virtual meetings are likely to continue and become popular alternatives to the regular 9–5 office jobs and face-to-face meetings due to the efficiencies and cost savings brought by these innovations. Similarly, online modes of delivering healthcare (telemedicine), financial services (bill payment, banking), entertainment (over-the-top or OTT, web streaming) have become ubiquitous ways to consume these services. For example, the demand for online medical appointments on Practo, a telehealth company in India, grew more than ten times between April and November 2020, and the company doubled its revenue in 2022 over 2021. These shifts to digital transactions have fueled an unforeseen growth in delivery, transportation, and warehouse jobs. For example, more than 5 million new jobs were created in the e-commerce, delivery, and social media businesses in China in the first half of 2020. COVID-19 has also led to faster adoption of emerging technologies (e.g., artificial intelligence) in jobs with high physical proximity.

3 COVID-19 early successes and failures

Battling the unknown

3.1 Testing, tracing, and isolation

One of the fundamental strategies in managing the pandemic was widespread testing, contact tracing, and isolation (Chung et al., 2021). Many countries established comprehensive testing regimes to identify cases early and isolate individuals to prevent further spread (Amir, 2022). South Korea and Singapore, for instance, implemented rigorous testing and contact tracing, utilizing technology to effectively track and contain outbreaks. COVID-19 testing, tracing, and isolation were essential components of public health strategies to control the spread of the COVID-19 virus. These measures aimed to identify and isolate infected individuals, trace their contacts, and provide timely medical care to those affected (Ashcroft et al., 2022).

Several types of COVID-19 tests were developed, including PCR (Polymerase Chain Reaction) tests, antigen tests, and antibody tests (Chau et al., 2020). *PCR tests:* PCR tests were the most commonly used and considered the gold standard. They detect the genetic material of the virus in a person's respiratory sample (usually from a nasal or throat swab). PCR tests are highly accurate but can take several hours to yield results. *Antigen tests:* Antigen tests were faster but less sensitive than PCR tests. They detect specific viral proteins and are often used for rapid screening. *Antibody tests:* Antibody tests detect antibodies produced by the body in response to the virus and useful to determine past infections but not for diagnosing active cases.

Most governments and health authorities also established protocols to slow down the spread of the virus with guidelines for contact tracing to identify close contacts and issue appropriate notifications. *Contact tracing:* Contact tracing involved identifying and notifying individuals who had close contact with someone who tested positive for COVID-19 virus. This was typically done by public health departments or contact tracing apps. *Close contacts:* Close contacts were people who had been within a certain proximity to an infected individual for a specified duration. The criteria for defining close contacts varied but often included household members, coworkers, and others who spent a significant amount of time together. *Notifications:* Close contacts were informed about their potential exposure to the virus and advised to self-quarantine, monitor for symptoms, and get tested. Contact tracers

DOI: 10.4324/9781003227113-4

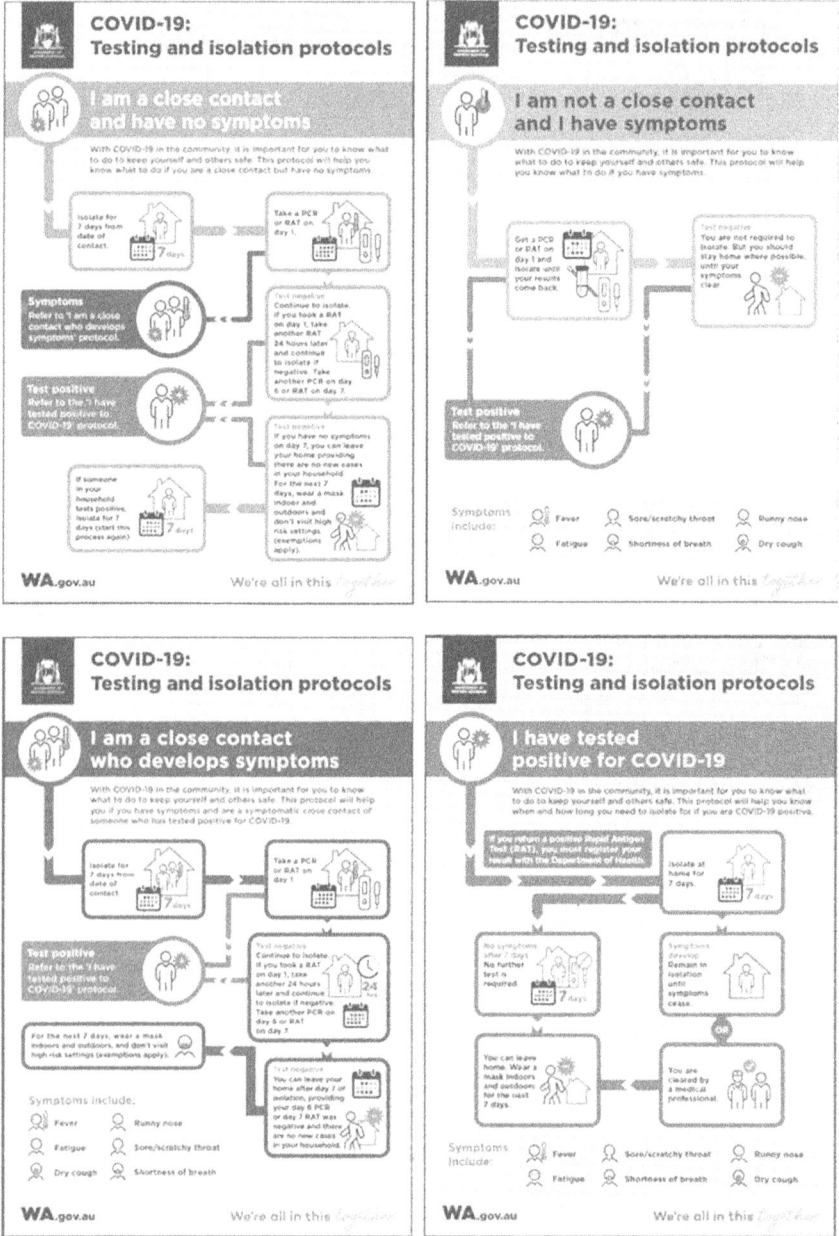

Figure 3.1 COVID-19 protocols for different types of cases

Source: Western Australian Government (http://wa.gov.au)

also collected information about the contacts' recent interactions to continue the chain of tracing if they tested positive. Figure 3.1 shows examples of COVID-19 protocols for different types of cases used in Western Australia.

The final stage in the process of managing the spread of COVID-19 virus consisted of isolation and quarantine protocols (Aronna et al., 2021). *Isolation of infected individuals:* Individuals who tested positive for COVID-19 virus were advised to isolate themselves from others to prevent further spread. Isolation typically involved staying at home or in a designated facility until they were no longer contagious, often for a specific duration or until they met certain criteria (e.g., no symptoms for a certain period). *Quarantine for close contacts:* Close contacts of infected individuals were usually asked to quarantine themselves, which means staying away from others to see if they develop symptoms. If they tested positive or developed symptoms during quarantine, they would then be isolated.

All these testing, tracing, and isolation measures were only effective in controlling the spread of the virus when implemented comprehensively and in conjunction with other preventive measures like mask-wearing, social distancing, and vaccination (Memon et al., 2021). The success of these strategies also depended on widespread testing availability, efficient contact tracing, and the cooperation of individuals in following isolation and quarantine guidelines (Aronna et al., 2021). Variations in how these measures were implemented and their effectiveness occurred in different regions and countries depended on their resources, healthcare infrastructures, and public compliances.

3.2   Lockdowns and restrictions on movement

Most governments imposed some degree of lockdowns and movement restrictions to curb the virus's transmission, especially during the early stages of the pandemic, ranging from partial lockdowns to complete stay-at-home orders, which were aimed at reducing person-to-person interactions (Koh, 2020). While these restrictions came with economic and social costs, they proved effective in slowing the virus's spread, as seen in countries like China and New Zealand. Lockdowns and movement restrictions were among the most significant and widely implemented public health measures to control the spread of COVID-19. These measures aimed to limit social and physical interactions among people, slow down the transmission of the virus, and prevent healthcare systems from becoming overwhelmed (Amer et al., 2021). The specifics of how lockdowns and movement restrictions were implemented varied from one place to another, but all of them had some or all of the following common elements.

Stay-at-home orders: People were often required to stay at home except for essential activities such as buying groceries, seeking medical care, or going to work if their job was deemed essential. Non-essential businesses and services were usually temporarily closed. *Travel restrictions:* Governments imposed restrictions on domestic and international travel. This included border closures, quarantine requirements for travelers, and limitations on the movement of people between regions or cities. *Closure of public spaces:* Public spaces such as parks, playgrounds, gyms, and recreational facilities were often closed to prevent gatherings and encourage social distancing. *School closures:* Educational institutions, from schools to universities, were closed to limit the spread of the virus among students and staff. Many institutions shifted to online learning (García-Morales et al., 2021). *Work-from-home policies:* Employers were encouraged or required to allow their employees to work from home whenever possible to reduce the number of people in workplaces.

Curfews: Some areas implemented curfews, restricting movement during certain hours of the day or night to discourage gatherings and socializing. *Mask mandates:* The use of face masks in public places became mandatory in many regions to reduce the transmission of the virus through respiratory droplets. *Enforcement:* Police and other authorities were tasked with enforcing these restrictions, often issuing fines or penalties to those who violated them. *Phased reopening:* As the situation improved, some areas adopted a phased approach to reopening, gradually relaxing restrictions on businesses, gatherings, and travel. *Monitoring and contact tracing:* Some countries implemented digital tools and contact tracing apps to monitor the spread of the virus and identify potential outbreaks. Figure 3.2 shows examples of COVID-19 announcements for getting in and out of lockdowns used in Western Australia.

It is important to note that the effectiveness and acceptance of these measures varied widely from place to place, and their implementation often depended on the severity of the COVID-19 outbreak in a particular region (Koh, 2020). Lockdowns and movement restrictions were controversial and had significant social and economic impacts, leading to debates about the balance between public health and individual freedoms (Williamson et al., 2021). Public health authorities continually monitored the situation and adjusted restrictions based on the evolving nature of the pandemic and vaccination efforts (Fu et al., 2022).

3.3   Quarantine, travel restrictions, and testing requirements

Many governments implemented quarantine and travel restrictions to contain imported cases and limit the virus's entry into their countries, including mandatory quarantine for travelers and border closures (Chu et al., 2020). For example, Australia's approach of strict border controls and mandatory quarantine for returning citizens helped the country to remain COVID-19 virus free for prolonged periods and to keep the number of cases and deaths significantly lower compared to other developed countries (Patel et al., 2020b). COVID-19 quarantine and travel restrictions were implemented by governments and health authorities worldwide mainly to limit the spread of the virus and protect public health. However, the specific details of these measures varied by country and region, with the following common characteristics.

Mandatory quarantine for infected individuals: Individuals who tested positive for COVID-19 virus or exhibited symptoms were often required to isolate themselves at home or in designated facilities until they were no longer contagious. The duration of isolation varied depending on local guidelines.

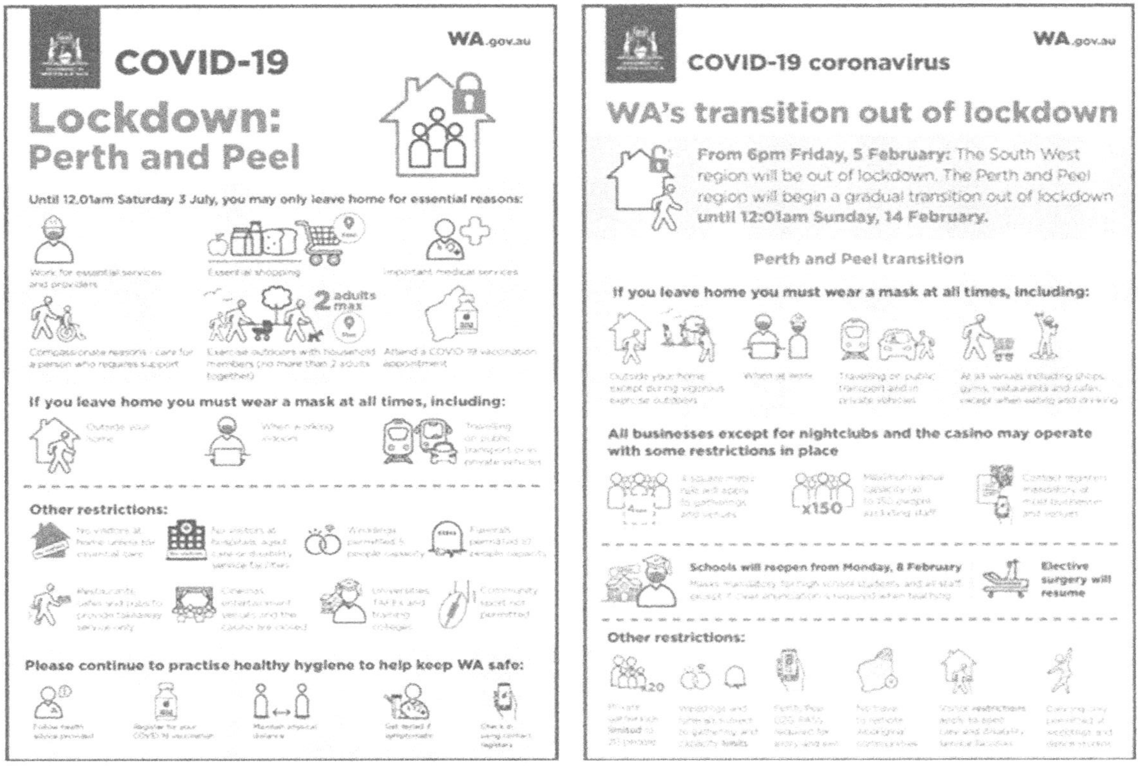

Figure 3.2 COVID-19 lockdown announcements in Western Australia

Source: Western Australian Government (http://wa.gov.au)

Quarantine for close contacts: People who had been in close contact with a confirmed COVID-19 case were often required to quarantine themselves for a specified period, usually from 10 to 14 days. This was done to prevent potential transmission if they were asymptomatic carriers. All these mandatory quarantine measures played an important role in controlling the initial spread of COVID-19. However, these were also found to be positively associated with a higher incidence of depression and emotional distress, perceived discrimination and risk of infection, as well as self-harm or suicidal intentions, especially in countries like China, with very strict implementation of these measures (Xin et al., 2020). Perceived discrimination was moderately and positively associated with emotional distress Therefore, it is very important to incorporate the mental health perspective into the planning and implementation of quarantine measures in future to minimize their negative impact. Figure 3.3 shows a comparison

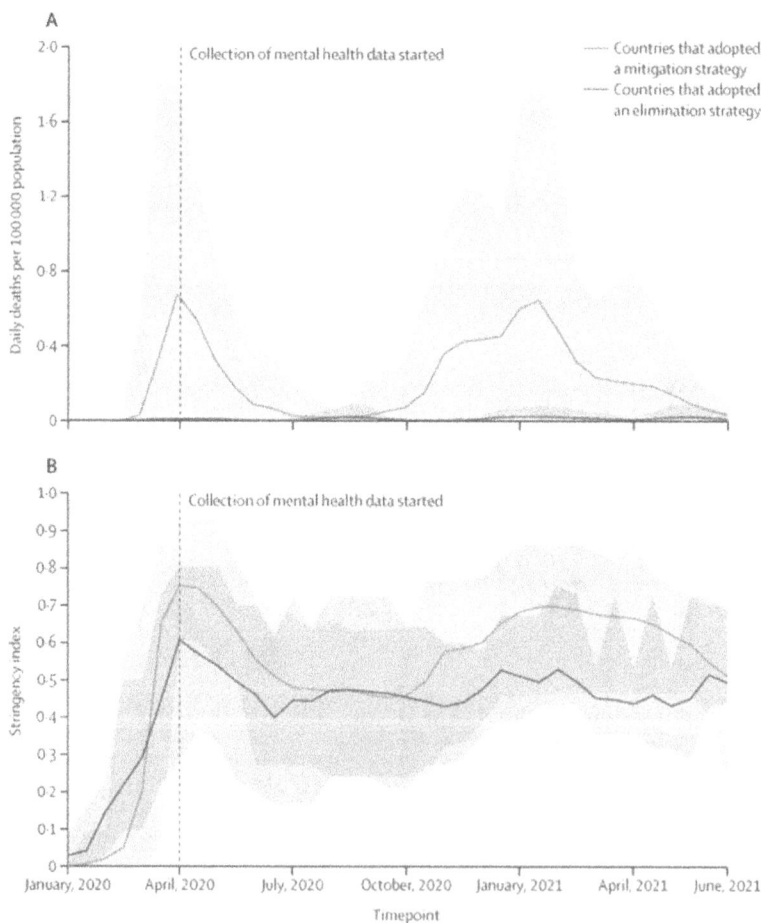

Figure 3.3 Comparison of pandemic intensity (A) and policy stringency (B)
Source: Aknin et al. (2022)

of pandemic intensity (A) and policy stringency (B) in 15 countries adopting a mix of mitigation and elimination strategies from April 2020 when the collection of mental health data started to June 2021 when the pandemic started slowing down around the world (Aknin et al., 2022).

International travel restrictions: Many countries imposed restrictions on international travel. These restrictions often included border closures, travel bans, or mandatory quarantine periods for travelers arriving from high-risk areas. Travelers were required to provide negative COVID-19 test results before or after their journeys. *Domestic travel restrictions:* Some regions within countries implemented travel restrictions between cities or regions with high infection rates and those with lower rates. Travel permits or documentation were sometimes required for intercity or interstate travel. *Travel bans:* Some countries imposed bans on travelers from specific countries or regions with high infection rates. These bans were frequently adjusted based on the evolving situation. While all these travel restrictions and bans gave a sense of security to the countries implementing these, World Health Organization (WHO) actually counseled against unilateral and outright travel bans as according to them, these restrictions could hamper the supplies and deliveries of much-needed medical aid, essential equipment, and technical support (Devi, 2020). Researchers also found that the travel restrictions to and from China only moderately affected the further spread of virus if it was already circulating in the community, and hence, early detection, hand washing, self-isolation, and household quarantine were more effective than travel restrictions to control further spread (Chinazzi et al., 2020).

Testing requirements: Travelers were often required to provide proof of a negative COVID-19 test before departure or upon arrival. Some places required both pre-departure and post-arrival testing. *Quarantine facilities:* Some countries provided designated facilities for quarantining travelers arriving from high-risk areas, especially if they did not have a suitable place to quarantine on their own. *Travel health declarations:* Travelers were often required to complete health declarations or questionnaires before traveling, disclosing their health status, recent travel history, and contact information. *Traveler monitoring:* Some countries implemented measures to monitor the health and whereabouts of travelers during their stay, such as mobile apps or daily check-ins. *Evacuation of citizens:* In some cases, governments organized the evacuation of their citizens from regions heavily affected by the virus, often requiring them to undergo quarantine upon their return. We must note that these measures were subject to change based on the evolving nature of the pandemic, the emergence of new variants, and vaccination efforts. Quarantine and travel restrictions were implemented to varying degrees of strictness and duration, depending on the severity of the COVID-19 outbreak in a given area and the public health policies of the local government. Travelers were advised to check with relevant authorities and follow local guidelines before planning their trips.

3.4   Public communication and awareness

Clear and consistent public communication was paramount in managing the pandemic. Governments used various channels to inform the public about preventive measures, guidelines, and updates on the virus (OECD, 2020a). For example, New Zealand Prime Minister Jacinda Ardern's empathetic communication style was lauded for fostering trust and adherence to public health guidelines. Social media also played a major role in communication and even miscommunication about the pandemic, including speculations about its origin, its symptoms, number of cases and deaths, vaccine availability and effectiveness, etc. (Ades, 2020). For example, social media platforms, such as Facebook and Twitter were used more frequently than traditional mass media, to share and seek essential information about the pandemic. An important lesson from this experience is that social media platforms can be used effectively and efficiently even in future, by healthcare authorities and other government agencies, to create awareness about other socially relevant messages. Figure 3.4 shows how public communication may be used to support policy and fight disinformation in future.

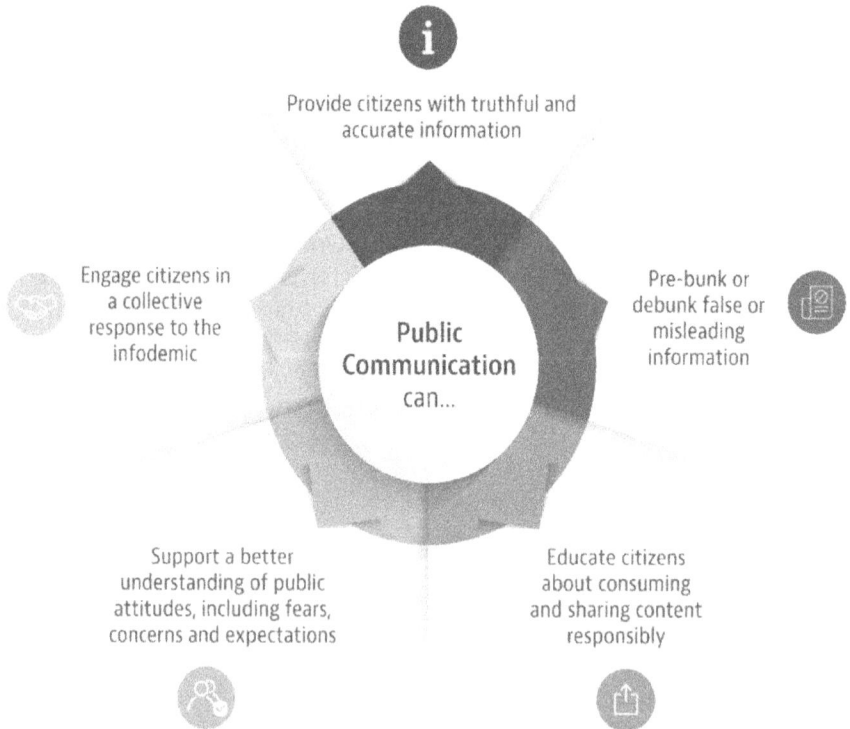

Provide citizens with truthful and accurate information

Engage citizens in a collective response to the infodemic

Public Communication can...

Pre-bunk or debunk false or misleading information

Support a better understanding of public attitudes, including fears, concerns and expectations

Educate citizens about consuming and sharing content responsibly

Figure 3.4 Using public communication to support policy and fight disinformation
Source: OECD

3.5 Economic stimulus packages

To mitigate the economic impact of lockdowns and reduce economic activity, governments implemented stimulus packages to support businesses, workers, and affected individuals. These measures aimed to prevent widespread job losses and business closures, such as the United States' Coronavirus Aid, Relief, and Economic Security (CARES) Act and Australia's Job Keeper programs. The CARES Act, was an unprecedented US$2.2 trillion economic stimulus bill passed by the 116th US Congress and signed into law by ex-President Donald Trump on 27 March 2020, aimed at helping the US economy recover from the economic impact of COVID-19. The spending included US$300 billion in one-time cash payments to individual taxpayers (with most single adults receiving $1,200 and families with children receiving more), US$260 billion in increased unemployment benefits, the creation of the Paycheck Protection Program that provided forgivable loans to small businesses with an initial US$350 billion in funding (later increased to US$669 billion by subsequent legislation), US$500 billion in loans for corporations, and US$340 billion to state and local governments (Taylor et al., 2020).

Similarly, the Australian government's JobKeeper Support Plan (Figure 3.5) costing about AUD$89 billion, helped keep Australians in jobs and supported businesses adversely affected by COVID-19. In the first phase (from 30 March to 27 September 2020), eligible businesses and not-for-profit organizations were able to receive AUD$1,500 (before tax) per fortnight per employee to

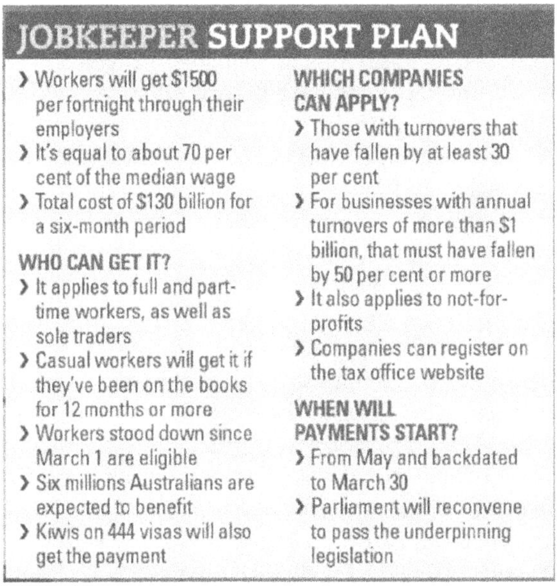

JOBKEEPER SUPPORT PLAN

- ❯ Workers will get $1500 per fortnight through their employers
- ❯ It's equal to about 70 per cent of the median wage
- ❯ Total cost of $130 billion for a six-month period

WHO CAN GET IT?
- ❯ It applies to full and part-time workers, as well as sole traders
- ❯ Casual workers will get it if they've been on the books for 12 months or more
- ❯ Workers stood down since March 1 are eligible
- ❯ Six millions Australians are expected to benefit
- ❯ Kiwis on 444 visas will also get the payment

WHICH COMPANIES CAN APPLY?
- ❯ Those with turnovers that have fallen by at least 30 per cent
- ❯ For businesses with annual turnovers of more than $1 billion, that must have fallen by 50 per cent or more
- ❯ It also applies to not-for-profits
- ❯ Companies can register on the tax office website

WHEN WILL PAYMENTS START?
- ❯ From May and backdated to March 30
- ❯ Parliament will reconvene to pass the underpinning legislation

Figure 3.5 Australia's JobKeeper Support plan

Source: Australian Taxation Office (www.ato.gov.au)

cover the cost of wages. This amount was scaled down during the next phase to AUD$1,200 per fortnight for employees who worked 20 hours or more a week and AUD$750 for employees who worked less than 20 hours a week on average from 28 September 2020 to 3 January 2021. Finally, the payment rate was reduced to AUD$1,000 per fortnight for employees who worked 20 hours or more a week and AUD$650 for employees who worked less than 20 hours a week on average from 4 January 2021 to 28 March 2021 period (Australian Treasury, 2023).

3.6   Remote work and digital solutions

In the early stages of COVID-19, the shift to remote work and digital solutions became crucial to maintain business continuity while minimizing physical interactions (Lund et al., 2021). Governments around the world implemented actions to support remote work and promote digital solutions during this time. These actions aimed at ensuring business continuity, reducing the spread of the virus, and supporting individuals and organizations in adapting to new ways of working. Countries with advanced digital infrastructure (e.g., Japan, Singapore, and South Korea) found themselves better prepared to implement remote work transitions and digital transformation of everyday activities. These government actions included the following:

Digital infrastructure investments: Many governments implemented policies and directives urging or mandating businesses to allow employees to work from home whenever possible to minimize physical contact and reduce the risk of transmission (Daneshfar et al., 2023). Some governments also provide financial support to businesses to help them invest in remote work infrastructure and technology, including grants, loans, or tax incentives. More importantly, most governments invested in improving digital infrastructure, such as upgrading broadband networks and expanding internet access in rural areas, to ensure reliable and high-speed connectivity for remote workers and students attending online classes at home (Strusani & Houngbonon, 2020). Similarly, many mobile applications were developed to help 'track and trace' the spread of the virus and researchers even used artificial intelligence (AI) to learn more about the virus and help with the efforts to search for a vaccine. With such an unprecedented increase in digital activity, it was not surprising to see the Internet traffic almost double in many countries shortly after the COVID-19 outbreak (OECD, 2020b). While these trends confirmed the huge potential for digital transformation, the pandemic also highlighted the digital divide, with people from the disadvantaged sections of the society unable to keep pace with others in terms of education, employment, health, and other important outcomes (OECD, 2020b).

Digital payments: COVID-19 also led to a dramatic jump in the use of digital payments, with over 40% of adults in low and middle-income economies (outside China) making in-store or online payments using a card, phone, or the internet and more than a third paying a utility bill directly from a formal account for the first time in their lives during COVID-19 (World Bank, 2022).

For example, more than 80 million adults in India and over 100 million in China made their first digital merchant payment after the start of the pandemic. In fact, two-thirds of adults worldwide now make or receive a digital payment, with the share in developing economies grew from 35% in 2014 to 57% in 2021. Similarly, 71% of adults in developing economies now have an account at a bank, other financial institution, or with a mobile money provider, up from 63% in 2017 and 42% in 2011. All these developments have led to greater financial inclusion in least-developed regions, such as Sub-Saharan Africa (World Bank, 2022).

Regulatory flexibility: Governments introduced temporary regulatory changes to facilitate remote work, such as easing restrictions on the use of digital signatures, allowing virtual meetings for official purposes, and relaxing data protection rules to enable smoother collaboration. For example, there was a critical urgency to develop and deliver effective vaccines and therapeutics, by speeding up ongoing clinical research, forming regulations, and ensuring supplies of necessary materials and facilities. European Commission, European Medicines Agency (EMA), and National Regulatory Agencies (NRAs) responded to this need by issuing guidance outlining regulatory flexibilities for COVID-19 vaccines and therapeutics (Klein et al., 2022). Research shows that digitalization was the key driver of these flexibilities along with innovations in regulatory process, such as rolling reviews and flexible scientific advice, which helped improve the overall process and outcomes (Klein et al., 2022).

Training and skill development: To help workers adapt to remote work, some governments initiated programs to provide training and skill development in digital tools and technologies, such as distance learning (Chun et al., 2021). Widespread business closures and losses in profits around the world during the early stages of COVID-19 had an adverse effect on opportunities for not only regular employment but also apprenticeship and internship positions. These were made worse by the lack of appropriate distance-learning platforms and educational resources, an almost complete break-down in the regular assessment and certification processes, and a steep drop in the motivation levels of learners and teachers alike due to all the anxiety, uncertainty, and economic hardship caused by the pandemic (Chun et al., 2021). However, notwithstanding these early setbacks, the development of flexible learning and assessment options through timely partnerships, new training programs and additional resources provided by the governments to overcome skills and labor shortages may prove to be a silver lining in future, by resulting in the emergence of innovative solutions in response to the pandemic.

Cybersecurity support: Besides its devastating impact on society and businesses as a whole, COVID-19 also led to unique circumstances that gave rise to cyber-crime opportunities, with the increased anxiety caused by the pandemic resulting in a greater number of cyber-attacks and hacking attempts (Lallie et al., 2021). Cyber-criminals preyed on specific events and governmental announcements in particular, to meticulously create and execute innovative cyber-crime campaigns. In response, governments collaborated with technology companies to develop and implement digital solutions for remote work, such as video conferencing tools, collaboration platforms, and pro-ject management software. Moreover, recognizing the increased reliance on digital platforms, governments took steps to enhance cybersecurity measures and provided guidance to businesses and individuals to protect against cyber threats associated with remote work (Lallie et al., 2021).

Overall, the specific actions taken by the governments to support remote work and digital transformation varied by country and region, depending on the severity of the pandemic and the existing infrastructure and policies in place. Moreover, these measures were often dynamic, with governments ad-justing their approaches based on the evolving nature of the pandemic.

3.7   International collaboration

International collaboration was crucial to understand the virus, share informa-tion, and coordinate efforts to control its spread during the early stages of the pandemic. Government agencies around the world collaborate with each other by sharing information, best practices, and research to develop vaccines and treatments (Liu et al., 2020). Initiatives like COVAX (led by Gavi, the Vaccine Alliance, the Coalition for Epidemic Preparedness Innovations (CEPI), and WHO) aimed to ensure equitable access to vaccines worldwide, acknowledging that global challenges demand collective solutions. Thus, COVID-19 forced governments worldwide to adopt a range of strategies to manage its impact. From testing and tracing to lockdowns, vaccination campaigns, and economic support, each strategy reflects the unique circumstances and priorities of indi-vidual countries. By showing no respect for national boundaries, COVID-19 has underscored the importance of flexibility, adaptability, and evidence-based decision-making, and emphasized the need for international collaboration to effectively address similar global crises in future using a systems approach to facilitate sharing of data and knowledge. For example, open access to standard-ized data required for globally regulated clinical research is essential to develop a global system to prevent and control future pandemics. However, it would not be easy due to challenges in combining data from different sources as they may follow a diverse range of formats and protocols (Ros et al., 2021).

Information sharing: Global health organizations, such as WHO, played a central role in collecting and disseminating information about the virus, its characteristics, and preventive measures (Tang et al., 2023). Throughout the pandemic, WHO facilitated communication among member countries and provided guidelines for response efforts, which were by and large followed by the member countries, although there was also a great deal of skepticism about the capabilities of WHO in anticipating and managing the pandemic (Bayram & Shields, 2021). Scientists and researchers from around the world collabo-rated to share data and findings using platforms like the Global Initiative on Sharing All Influenza Data (GISAID) that allowed scientists to share genomic data about the virus, which in turn was crucial to understanding its evolution and to develop diagnostic tools. Countries also collaborated on monitoring the spread of the virus through international surveillance systems to track and share the progression of the virus, identify hotspots, and implement timely interventions, to enable a coordinated response (Tang et al., 2023).

Development and distribution of medical resources: International collaboration played a critical role in the development of vaccines, with scientists, pharmaceutical companies, and governments from different countries working together to accelerate vaccine research, share data, and conduct clinical trials (Lee & Haupt, 2021). Countries with more resources supported those facing shortages by sharing medical supplies, personal protective equipment (PPE), and other essential resources. This collaborative effort aimed to ensure that all nations had the necessary tools to respond to the health crisis, highlighting the importance of international research collaboration to overcome the regional imbalances in the availability and access to knowledge across multiple inter-related disciplines (Kim & Cho, 2021). A review of research on coronavirus during the first few months of COVID-19 showed the prevalence of smaller teams and fewer nations (led by the US and China) than pre-COVID-19 period (Fry et al., 2020). Hence, it seems that the global COVID-19 pandemic shifted the geographic focus of coronavirus research and the structure of scientific teams with narrower and elite memberships. These findings raise important questions about the challenges scientists are likely to face in forming effective and efficient teams to rapidly respond to similar health crises in future.

Policy coordination: International organizations held regular meetings and conferences to coordinate global responses and share best practices, including discussions on testing strategies, treatment protocols, and public health measures. Many countries also aligned their policies and guidelines with international recommendations to create a more standardized approach to pandemic response and facilitate smoother collaboration. Most countries also coordinated their travel restrictions and guidelines to prevent the international spread of the virus by sharing information about infection rates, implementing quarantine measures, and updating travel advisories. International collaboration was also crucial to maintain the flow of essential goods, including medical supplies and food, by addressing disruptions in global supply chains. However, significant challenges were faced due to many countries choosing to follow their own priorities rather than joining other countries in developing a coordinated response to tackle the pandemic (Liu et al., 2021). For example, the Chinese government relied on vertical steering and horizontal support with strict controls on the movement of people outside their homes throughout the pandemic, the US government did not follow a single nationwide strategy and allowed all the states to devise and implement their own strategies. Despite these significant differences in national strategies, it is clear that effective multi-level governance in crisis responses requires a harmonious balance between centralized national leadership and local autonomy coupled with broader social engagement (Liu et al., 2021).

Financial support and assistance: Various countries and international organizations provided financial aid and support to nations severely affected by the pandemic, which helped them strengthen their healthcare systems and mitigate the economic impact of the crisis. Diplomatic efforts were also employed to foster international cooperation by engaging in diplomatic dialogues to address challenges, promote collaboration, and share insights on managing the pandemic. While there were instances of successful international collaboration, challenges also emerged, including vaccine distribution disparities, and geopolitical tensions, affecting information sharing, and issues related to equitable access to resources. Nevertheless, the global response to COVID-19 highlighted the importance of collaborative efforts in addressing a shared global health crisis, such as public awareness programs, testing and quarantining policies, and income support packages, due to their significant impact on the health of financial markets and stock market returns that are crucial to maintain economic health (Ashraf, 2020).

3.8   Vaccine development and communication campaigns

As vaccines became available, governments globally launched massive vaccination campaigns to achieve herd immunity and prevent severe cases. Different countries adopted varying strategies for vaccine distribution, targeting frontline workers, vulnerable populations, and the general public. Israel's rapid and widespread vaccination campaign served as a model for efficiently administering vaccines. International collaboration during vaccine development and communication campaigns was essential to ensure a coordinated and effective global response to the COVID-19 as it emphasized the importance of showing solidarity in addressing a shared global health challenge.

Vaccine development: Global scientific collaboration was key to tackling COVID-19 through rapid development of vaccines and this was facilitated by sharing research and data by scientists and researchers worldwide. Collaborations through international organizations, academic institutions, and platforms (e.g., GISAID) facilitated rapid exchange of information on the virus's genetic makeup and characteristics. WHO played a central role in coordinating global efforts by establishing tools, such as Access to COVID-19 Tools (ACTs) Accelerator, which helped accelerate the development, production, and equitable access to COVID-19 tests, treatments, and vaccines. Many countries also participated in global initiatives, such as COVAX, which aimed to ensure fair and equitable access to vaccines worldwide. Governments and international organizations also actively collaborated with pharmaceutical companies to expedite vaccine development, through greater research funding, clinical trials, and agreements for vaccine production and distribution.

Many global collaborative initiatives, such as CEPI provided funding for vaccine research and development, and encouraged cross-sector collaboration. CEPI is an innovative global partnership among public, private, philanthropic, and civil society organizations, working together to accelerate the development of vaccines against emerging infectious diseases and to enable equitable access to these vaccines for people during any future pandemic (www.cepi.net/). Countries also worked to harmonize regulatory processes to accelerate vaccine approvals. Many regulatory agencies collaborated closely to share information and ensure that rigorous safety and efficacy standards were met (Bolislis et al., 2021). Some countries implemented expedited approval processes, such as emergency use authorizations, to allow the use of vaccines in the early stages of development (Tran & Witek, 2021).

Communication campaigns: WHO provided guidelines and recommendations for communication strategies, emphasizing the importance of clear and consistent messaging, to ensure that information about the virus, vaccines, and preventive measures was communicated accurately (WHO, 2020). Most countries participated in global public health campaigns to promote preventive measures such as mask-wearing, hand hygiene, and social distancing, which were often followed as internationally recognized guidelines (Curtis et al., 2020). Many countries also coordinated their public communication efforts to provide consistent messaging on vaccine safety, efficacy, and distribution plans (Noar & Austin, 2020). This coordination aimed to build public trust and address misinformation. Governments collaborated with international media outlets to disseminate accurate information and counter misinformation related to vaccines. Countries also aimed to ensure equitable access to messaging by participating in platforms like COVAX by sharing information about vaccine distribution plans and addressing concerns related to vaccine nationalism. Attempts were also made to engage the communities through community outreach programs to address vaccine hesitancy, educate the public about the importance of vaccination, and dispel myths and misinformation. Communication campaigns were also designed to be inclusive, considering cultural and linguistic diversity to reach different populations effectively (Colleoni et al., 2022).

3.9   Conclusion

The early successes and failures in combating COVID-19 have illuminated the complexities of managing a global pandemic. Effective responses hinged on proactive measures, robust healthcare systems, transparent communication, and international collaboration. The lessons learned from the early stages of the pandemic provide a roadmap for nations to better navigate future crises and work collectively toward global health security. For example, swift and stringent lockdowns and travel restrictions by countries like New Zealand, Australia, and South Korea in the early stages of the pandemic, helped them effectively control the virus's spread. These measures allowed these nations to contain the virus, prevent overwhelming healthcare systems, and protect vulnerable populations. Similarly, countries like Germany and Taiwan showcased effective communication strategies, including transparent dissemination of accurate information, clear guidelines, and timely updates that bolstered public trust and compliance with preventive measures, which helped them control the initial spread of the virus. Aggressive testing and contact tracing during the early stages of the pandemic also played a pivotal role in identifying and isolating infected individuals in a proactive manner to curb the initial transmission rates and prevent large-scale outbreaks. Finally, in countries like Vietnam, community engagement and mobilization were instrumental in disseminating information, promoting hygiene practices, and facilitating compliance with public health guidelines.

On the flip side, there are important lessons to be learned from the early failures in the battle against COVID-19. For example, many nations faced criticism for delayed responses to the pandemic, such as delayed lockdowns and inadequate testing during the initial stages, which allowed the virus to spread unchecked, leading to higher infection rates and putting tremendous strains on their healthcare systems subsequently. Similarly, countries with limited healthcare infrastructure struggled to cope with the surge in cases due to insufficient hospital beds, ventilators, and medical supplies, which hindered their ability to provide critical care to patients, resulting in higher mortality rates. Balancing public health measures with political and economic considerations also posed challenges for some governments (e.g., US), resulting in delayed lockdowns and premature opening, which led to subsequent waves of infections, prolonging the pandemic's impact. The spread of misinformation and disinformation further impeded effective response to the pandemic as inaccurate information eroded public trust, leading to non-compliance with preventive measures and hindering contact tracing efforts. Next, we discuss a few important lessons for managers from the early successes and failures that the world experienced in the global battle with the pandemic during its early stages.

3.10   Future lessons for managers

The early successes and failures in the fight against COVID-19 offer valuable lessons for future pandemic preparedness. First and foremost, it highlighted the importance of proactive and decisive actions in the early stages of any crisis, as we saw the crucial role that swift, decisive, and evidence-based actions could have played in containing the virus's spread and preventing overwhelming healthcare systems. Second, being prepared through capacity building by investing in robust infrastructure and other resources, including data, knowledge, people, processes, and systems, is equally essential to effectively manage any crisis and provide an adequate and proportionate response. Third, we highlight the importance of transparent, clear, and consistent communication to build public trust, promote compliance, and counter misinformation, in any crisis internal or external to any organization. Finally, the early global responses to COVID-19 underline the importance of greater international cooperation, with collaborative efforts, data sharing, and knowledge exchange across nations, to develop effective containment strategies and accelerate vaccine development. We recommend managers acknowledge and accept the importance of these lessons in not only anticipating and managing external crises such as COVID-19, but also internal crises that they may face from time to time, such as product failures, loss in staff morale, and any other adverse events.

4 COVID-19 subsequent waves and new strains

Living with the enemy

4.1 Subsequent waves

Subsequent waves of COVID-19 refer to surges in cases that occurred after the initial outbreak has been brought under control or stabilized. The experiences and impacts of the second wave of COVID-19 varied across different regions and countries in their intensity, duration, and geographic scope. The timing, severity, and specific events during the second wave depended on factors such as public health measures implemented, healthcare system capacity, population density, and the effectiveness of containment efforts. Specifically, the timing of the second wave varied globally, with some regions experiencing it in late 2020, while others faced it in early 2021. In some areas, the second wave was more severe than the initial wave, leading to increased numbers of cases, hospitalizations, and deaths, such as in India (Malik, 2022). During the second wave, several new variants of the SARS-CoV-2 virus were identified, which were often associated with changes in the virus's spike protein and, in some cases, increased transmissibility (Scandurra et al., 2023; Wetherall et al., 2022).

It's important to note that the situation during the second wave varied widely, and different regions faced unique challenges (Amer et al., 2022; Malik, 2022). The dynamics of subsequent waves, including the emergence of new variants and vaccination progress, continued to shape the global response to the ongoing COVID-19 pandemic (Girardi et al., 2022). For the most current and region-specific information, it was recommended to consult reputable health authorities and official government sources. Several factors contribute to the occurrence of subsequent waves, including the relaxation of measures, such as easing of lockdowns, removal of travel restrictions, and social distancing measures, which led to increased transmission as people began to interact more freely (Wei et al., 2022). The emergence of new variants and levels of immunity in the population also influenced the timing and severity of subsequent waves. Some respiratory viruses, like coronaviruses, also exhibit seasonality, with increased transmission during specific seasons, like winter. The rate of vaccination and the effectiveness of vaccines can also impact the likelihood and impact of subsequent waves. All these factors led to many changes in the

DOI: 10.4324/9781003227113-5

impact of COVID-19 and the strategies used by governments and businesses around the world to restrict its further spread (Liu et al., 2022; Malik, 2022; Wei et al., 2022), as described in detail in this section.

4.1.1   *Impact on healthcare systems*

Healthcare systems faced increased strain, with hospitals experiencing surges in COVID-19 patients. Some areas reported shortages of medical supplies, ventilators, and healthcare personnel. Intensive care units (ICUs) in some regions operated at or near full capacity (Hartley & Perencevich, 2020; Hobin & Smith, 2020). Many countries implemented or reinforced public health measures during the second wave. These measures included lockdowns, social distancing, mask mandates, and restrictions on gatherings. Governments and health authorities emphasized the importance of hand hygiene and encouraged the use of face masks to curb the spread of the virus. COVID-19 strained healthcare systems in several ways, and the impact varied across regions based on factors such as the severity of the outbreak, healthcare infrastructure, and the effectiveness of public health measures, as discussed in this section.

Surge in hospitalizations: COVID-19 led to a significant increase in the number of patients requiring hospitalization, especially those with severe respiratory symptoms. The sudden surge in hospital admissions strained existing bed capacities and overwhelmed healthcare facilities (Hartley & Perencevich, 2020). *ICU overload:* Patients with severe cases of COVID-19 often require intensive care, including mechanical ventilation. The demand for ICU beds, ventilators, and critical care staff exceeded available resources in many areas (Tulenko & Vervoort, 2020). *Shortages of medical supplies:* The increased demand for medical supplies, including personal protective equipment (PPE), ventilators, and medications, led to shortages. Healthcare workers face challenges in accessing essential protective gear, putting them at risk of infection (Kirk & Mitchell, 2023). *Healthcare worker fatigue and burnout:* Healthcare workers faced immense physical and emotional stress due to the high volume of COVID-19 cases, long working hours, and emotionally challenging nature of the pandemic. Burnout and fatigue became prevalent issues (Hobin & Smith, 2020).

Redirection of resources: Hospitals had to redirect resources and personnel to address the influx of COVID-19 patients. This often meant postponing elective surgeries and other non-urgent medical procedures to prioritize resources for pandemic response (Sharma et al., 2021). *Supply chain disruptions:* The global nature of the pandemic disrupted supply chains for medical equipment and pharmaceuticals. Some regions experienced shortages of critical supplies due to increased demand and transportation disruptions (Panwar et al., 2022; Spieske & Birkel, 2021). *Challenges in testing and diagnosis:* The need for widespread testing placed a strain on laboratory capacities, leading to delays in test results, thus identifying and diagnosing COVID-19 cases became a logistical challenge (Moosavi et al., 2022).

Adaptation to new protocols: Healthcare systems had to rapidly adapt to new protocols for managing COVID-19 patients, including infection prevention and control measures, isolation procedures, and treatment protocols. This required additional training and resources. ***Impact on non-COVID-19 care:*** The focus on managing COVID-19 cases often resulted in delays or disruptions in the delivery of non-COVID-19 healthcare services. Patients with chronic conditions or those in need of routine care faced challenges in accessing medical services. ***Financial strain on healthcare institutions:*** The costs associated with managing the pandemic, including increased staffing, acquiring additional equipment, and implementing safety measures, placed financial strain on healthcare institutions, particularly those in already resource-constrained settings (Maani & Galea, 2020). All these strains on the healthcare systems highlighted the importance of robust preparedness, the need for surge capacity planning, and the significance of international collaboration in responding to global health crises. The ongoing efforts to mitigate the impact include vaccination campaigns, public health measures, and ongoing research to improve treatment protocols (Hartley & Perencevich, 2020).

4.1.2 Launch of vaccine campaigns

The second wave marked the early stages of COVID-19 vaccination campaigns in several countries. Vaccination efforts aimed to protect vulnerable populations, reduce severe illness and mortality, and contribute to achieving herd immunity although some regions faced challenges in vaccine distribution, availability, and equitable access. The launch of COVID-19 vaccine campaigns marked a significant milestone in the global effort to control the pandemic (Lee & Haupt, 2021). Vaccination campaigns were initiated to protect populations from severe illness, reduce hospitalizations and deaths, and contribute to achieving herd immunity. In this section, we provide an overview of the launch and impact of COVID-19 vaccine campaigns.

Vaccine development and approval: The rapid development of COVID-19 vaccines was facilitated by advancements in vaccine technology, global collaboration among scientists, and unprecedented funding and resources. Regulatory agencies in different countries conducted thorough reviews of vaccine candidates to ensure safety and efficacy (Klein et al., 2022). ***Emergency use authorizations:*** Some countries granted emergency use authorizations to expedite the deployment of vaccines before full regulatory approval, especially during the early stages of the pandemic (Liu et al., 2020). ***Global distribution:*** Vaccines were distributed globally via many mechanisms, including bilateral agreements between countries, multilateral initiatives, and collaborations with international organizations (Sharma et al., 2020).

Phased rollout: Most countries implemented phased rollout plans, prioritizing high-risk populations, such as healthcare workers, the elderly, and individuals with underlying health conditions, in the initial stages (WHO, 2020). ***Logistics and cold chain management:*** Cold chain management became crucial to ensure the integrity of the vaccines during transportation and storage as the distribution of vaccines presented logistical challenges, especially for vaccines with specific temperature storage requirements (Klobucista, 2022). *Public communication and education:* Governments and health organizations engaged in extensive public communication campaigns to educate the public about the importance of vaccination, address concerns, and combat misinformation. *Vaccine administration:* Vaccination centers were set up, ranging from large-scale vaccination sites to mobile clinics, to administer doses efficiently. Some countries also utilize existing healthcare infrastructure, pharmacies, and community clinics for vaccination (Libotte et al., 2020; Thye et al., 2021).

4.1.3 *Impact of COVID-19 vaccine campaigns*

The impact of COVID-19 vaccine campaigns has been substantial in reducing the severity of the disease and contributing to the global effort to bring the pandemic under control (Cadeddu et al., 2022; Wang et al., 2022a). However, ongoing efforts are needed to achieve widespread vaccination coverage and address evolving challenges in the fight against COVID-19 (Dhama et al., 2021; WHO, 2022). In this section, we discuss the various aspects of how Covid-19 vaccine campaigns have affected not only the spread of virus but also how people, organizations, and governments have responded to the dynamic changes associated with it.

Reduction in severe cases and hospitalizations: Vaccination campaigns contributed to a significant reduction in severe cases of COVID-19, leading to fewer hospitalizations and admissions to ICUs (Charitos et al., 2022). *Decrease in mortality rates:* Vaccination played a crucial role in lowering mortality rates, particularly among older populations and individuals with underlying health conditions who were at higher risk of severe outcomes (He et al., 2022). *Easing of public health measures:* Successful vaccination campaigns led to the gradual easing of certain public health measures, such as lockdowns and restrictions, as vaccination coverage increased and the risk of severe disease diminished (Cadeddu et al., 2022). *Impact on transmission:* Vaccination campaigns had a positive impact on reducing the transmission of the virus within communities and contributing to the overall control of the pandemic (Wang et al., 2022a).

Boosters and variants response: As new variants of the virus emerged, booster dose campaigns were initiated in various countries to enhance immunity and address concerns about waning vaccine effectiveness (Shah & Coiado, 2023). *Global efforts for equitable access:* Initiatives like COVAX aimed to ensure equitable access to vaccines globally, with a focus on providing doses to low- and middle-income countries (Roozen et al., 2022). *Challenges and variability:* Challenges included vaccine hesitancy, supply chain disruptions, and logistical complexities. Vaccine distribution and coverage varied widely between countries and regions (Sparke & Levy, 2022). *Ongoing surveillance and adaptation:* Ongoing surveillance, research, and monitoring of vaccine effectiveness were critical in adapting strategies to address emerging challenges, including new variants of the virus (Dhama et al., 2021; WHO, 2022).

4.1.4 *Economic impact*

The second wave also had economic consequences, with disruptions to businesses, travel, and various industries caused by continued lockdowns and restrictions implemented to control the spread of the virus (Wang et al., 2023). The economic impact of the second wave of COVID-19 varied across regions and countries, depending on factors such as the severity of the outbreak, the effectiveness of public health measures, and the resilience of the local economy. The economic impact of the second wave was intertwined with public health outcomes, vaccination progress, and the effectiveness of policy responses (Zaki et al., 2022). The situation evolved dynamically, and ongoing efforts to manage the pandemic, support affected sectors, and promote economic recovery continued in subsequent waves and phases of the COVID-19 pandemic (WEF, 2022). This section describes some trends and impacts associated with the economic consequences of the second wave.

Disruptions to businesses: Lockdowns, restrictions on movement, and social distancing measures implemented during the second wave had significant effects on businesses. Many sectors, especially hospitality, tourism, and non-essential retail, experienced disruptions and revenue losses (Delardas et al., 2022). *Employment and labor market:* The second wave led to job losses and increased unemployment in certain sectors directly impacted by restrictions. This included workers in industries such as hospitality, entertainment, and travel (Cortes & Forsythe, 2023; Villarreal & Yu, 2022). *Supply chain disruptions:* Restrictions and lockdowns affected global and regional supply chains, leading to disruptions in the production and distribution of goods. Some industries faced challenges in sourcing raw materials and components, resulting in delays and shortages (Moosavi et al., 2022; Ozdemir et al., 2022).

Impact on small businesses: Small and medium-sized enterprises (SMEs), which often have fewer resources to weather economic downturns, faced particular challenges. Many struggled to stay afloat due to reduced demand, operational restrictions, and financial constraints (Dejardin et al., 2023). *Financial markets and investor confidence:* Financial markets experienced volatility as investors reacted to uncertainties associated with the second wave and its potential economic impacts. Changes in investor confidence influenced stock prices and other financial indicators (Dietrich et al., 2022). *Government fiscal measures:* Governments implemented fiscal measures to mitigate the economic impact of the second wave. These measures included financial aid packages, stimulus programs, and support for affected industries and individuals (World Bank, 2020). *Increased debt levels:* Many governments increased their levels of public debt to finance economic stimulus packages and support measures. This raised concerns about the long-term fiscal sustainability and the need for future debt management (Augustin et al., 2022).

Digital transformation acceleration: The second wave accelerated the adoption of digital technologies as businesses and individuals adapted to remote work, online shopping, and virtual communication. This digital transformation had both positive and negative effects on different sectors (World

Bank, 2022). *Inflationary pressures:* Supply chain disruptions and increased government spending contributed to inflationary pressures in some regions. Rising inflation affected consumer purchasing power and impacted overall economic stability (De Soyres et al., 2022). *Vaccine rollout and economic optimism:* The rollout of COVID-19 vaccines during the second wave brought hope for economic recovery (Klobucista, 2022). Countries with successful vaccination campaigns saw improvements in economic sentiment and some restrictions were gradually lifted (Shah & Coiado, 2023).

4.1.5 Government responses

Governments adjusted their strategies based on lessons learned from the initial wave with response measures tailored to the specific circumstances and needs of each region (Liu et al., 2022). Communication efforts focused on providing clear and timely information to the public about the evolving situation and the importance of adhering to public health guidelines (Sauer et al., 2021). Government responses to the second wave of COVID-19 varied widely across countries and regions, with the nature and intensity of these responses influenced by many factors, such as the severity of the outbreak, healthcare infrastructure, vaccination status, and the economic and social context (Scandurra et al., 2023). The effectiveness of these measures varied and governments often adjusted their strategies based on the evolving situation and as a result, the balance between public health and economic considerations remained a complex challenge for policymakers during the second wave of the COVID-19 pandemic (Stobart & Duckett, 2022). This section describes government responses during the second wave.

Reimposition of public health measures: Governments reintroduced or reinforced public health measures, including lockdowns, social distancing, mask mandates, and restrictions on gatherings, to curb the spread of the virus (Stobart & Duckett, 2022). *Vaccination campaign intensification:* During the second wave, most governments intensified COVID-19 vaccination campaigns, including expanding eligibility criteria, increasing vaccine distribution, setting up additional vaccination centers, and addressing vaccine hesitancy (Amer et al., 2022). *Testing and contact tracing:* Increased testing capacity and efficient contact tracing were prioritized to identify and isolate cases promptly with widespread testing campaigns to identify and isolate cases rapidly (Amer et al., 2022). *Healthcare system support:* Governments provided additional support to healthcare systems, including the recruitment of healthcare workers, expansion of hospital capacity, and the procurement of medical supplies and equipment (Sharma et al., 2021). *Travel restrictions and border controls:* Travel restrictions and border controls were implemented again and further extended to limit the movement of people and reduce the risk of importing and exporting COVID-19 cases. Quarantine measures for travelers were often enforced (Stobart & Duckett, 2022). *Communication and public awareness:* Governments engaged in extensive communication campaigns to inform the public about the severity of the second wave, the importance of following public health guidelines, and the benefits of vaccination (Liu et al., 2022).

Economic support measures: Governments introduced or extended economic support measures to assist individuals and businesses affected by the second wave. This included financial aid, subsidies, and stimulus packages (Augustin et al., 2022). *Education adaptations:* Education systems underwent adaptations, with some regions implementing remote learning, hybrid models, or temporary closures of schools and universities to reduce the risk of transmission (Mittal et al., 2022). *Targeted lockdowns and restrictions:* Rather than implementing blanket lockdowns, some governments opted for targeted measures, such as localized lockdowns in areas with high infection rates or restrictions on specific types of businesses or events (Stobart & Duckett, 2022). *International cooperation:* Governments collaborate with international organizations and neighboring countries to share information, resources, and best practices. This cooperation aimed to address common challenges and facilitate a unified global response (Kim & Cho, 2021). *Accelerated vaccine approvals:* Some regions expedited the approval processes for new vaccines or booster shots to enhance their vaccination strategies in response to emerging variants and concerns about waning immunity (Klobucista, 2022). *Community engagement and support:* Community engagement and support programs were implemented to address pandemic fatigue and mental health concerns as well as to foster a sense of solidarity among the population (Scandurra et al., 2023).

4.1.6 Community fatigue and mental health

The second wave of the COVID-19 pandemic brought about significant challenges related to community fatigue and mental health issues. Communities experienced pandemic fatigue as prolonged periods of uncertainty, isolation, and economic challenges took a toll on mental health, while governments and health organizations continued to emphasize the importance of mental health support and community resilience (Bullock et al., 2022; Scandurra et al., 2023). Addressing mental health issues during the second wave and beyond required a comprehensive and community-centered approach, including increased access to mental health services, destigmatization of mental health discussions, and community-driven support mechanisms (Wetherall et al., 2022), as discussed in this section.

Prolonged uncertainty: The prolonged nature of the pandemic, with the emergence of subsequent waves, created an environment of ongoing uncertainty. This uncertainty, coupled with the dynamic nature of the situation, contributed to heightened stress and anxiety within communities (Sharma et al., 2020). *Cumulative impact of multiple waves:* Communities were already dealing with the repercussions of the initial wave of COVID-19 when subsequent waves hit. The cumulative impact of multiple waves, each with its own set of challenges and uncertainties, added to the mental health burden on individuals and communities (Scandurra et al., 2023). *Continued social isolation:* Lockdowns, social distancing measures, and restrictions on gatherings persisted during the second wave. The continued social isolation and limited face-to-face interactions took a toll on people's mental well-being, contributing to feelings of loneliness and isolation (Williams et al., 2021). ***Grief and loss:*** The second wave often brought an increase in the number of infections, hospitalizations, and deaths. Communities experienced collective grief and loss, whether directly through the illness or death of loved ones or indirectly through the impact on the community as a whole (Kumar, 2023).

Economic strain: Economic challenges resulting from the pandemic, such as job losses, financial insecurity, and business closures, exacerbated stress and anxiety within communities. The economic strain was particularly felt by individuals and families already facing financial difficulties (Augustin et al., 2022). ***Disruption to daily lives:*** Ongoing disruptions to daily life, including changes in work routines, remote learning, and limitations on recreational activities, contributed to a sense of upheaval. These disruptions affected the overall well-being of individuals and families (El-Shabasy et al., 2022). ***Healthcare worker burnout:*** Healthcare workers, who were at the forefront of the response to the pandemic, experienced heightened levels of stress and burnout during the second wave. The increased workload, emotional toll, and constant exposure to critical situations took a toll on their mental health (Balser et al., 2021). ***Pandemic fatigue:*** Many individuals and communities experienced pandemic fatigue, characterized by a sense of weariness and decreased motivation to adhere to public health guidelines resulting in a lack of compliance with preventive measures, which in turn could have further contributed to spread of the virus (Scandurra et al., 2023).

Impact on vulnerable populations: Vulnerable populations, including those with pre-existing mental health conditions, individuals living alone, and marginalized communities, faced heightened challenges during the second wave as they often had fewer resources and support systems to cope with the additional stressors (Malik, 2022). ***Need for mental health support:*** The increased recognition of mental health challenges during the pandemic underscored the need for accessible mental health support services. Governments, organizations, and communities worked to expand mental health resources and promote awareness of available services (Wetherall et al., 2022). ***Community resilience and support:*** Despite the challenges, communities also demonstrated resilience and solidarity. Support networks, community initiatives, and mental health outreach programs emerged to provide assistance and foster a sense of connection (Fransen et al., 2022; Yi et al., 2023).

4.2   New strains and variants

The SARS-CoV-2 virus has displayed a propensity for genetic mutation, resulting in the emergence of new strains and variants, including Alpha, Beta, Gamma, Delta, and Omicron (Jacobs et al., 2023). All these variants differ in terms of transmissibility, severity of illness, and potential impact on immunity, and show many unique features, including greater transmissibility, vaccine resistance, and unpredictable nature. Each variant has unique genetic mutations in the spike protein or other regions of the virus (El-Shabasy et al., 2022). These mutations can impact various characteristics of the virus, such as transmissibility, severity of illness, and potentially its ability to evade immunity generated by previous infection or vaccination (Hebbani et al., 2022). Variants are a natural part of virus evolution, and scientists continuously study their impact on the course of the pandemic and the effectiveness of preventive measures and vaccines (McLean et al., 2022). Hence, it is essential to monitor ongoing research and updates from health authorities, as new variants may emerge, and additional information on existing variants may become available.

Greater transmissibility: Some variants, like the Delta variant, are more transmissible than earlier strains. This can lead to faster and more extensive outbreaks. *Vaccine resistance:* Variants may have different levels of resistance to immunity acquired through vaccination or previous infection. Booster shots and modified vaccines may be necessary to address these challenges. *Unpredictable nature:* Surveillance and monitoring of variants are critical to understanding their prevalence and impact. Early detection allows for rapid response and containment measures. Each variant may have unique features, including specific genetic mutations that distinguish it from the original virus. Although ongoing research may reveal additional insights, Table 4.1 shows the main COVID-19 variants and mutants identified so far.

Table 4.1 Unique features of new strains and variants

Variant	First identified	Key mutations	Characteristics
Alpha variant (B.1.1.7)	United Kingdom (September 2020)	N501Y, P681H, and others	Associated with higher transmissibility and increased severity compared to earlier strains, including increased risk of severe illness.
Beta variant (B.1.351)	South Africa (May 2020)	E484K, N501Y, and others	Higher concerns about the reduced effectiveness of certain vaccines, particularly in preventing infection and increased transmissibility.
Gamma variant (P.1)	Brazil (November 2020)	E484K, N501Y, and others	Increased transmissibility and the E484K mutation in particular raised concerns about immune escape, including reinfections.
Delta variant (B.1.617.2)	India (October 2020)	L452R, T478K, and others	Became dominant strain in many regions due to its enhanced transmissibility and risk of hospitalization due to increased severity and potential adverse impact on vaccine effectiveness.
Omicron variant (B.1.1.529)	Southern Africa (November 2021)	N501Y, K417N, and others	Multiple mutations in the spike protein raised concerns about higher transmissibility, immune escape, and lower vaccine effectiveness.

Source: Compiled by authors from diverse sources on the Internet.

4.3   Implications for public health

Subsequent waves and new variants of COVID-19 present several implications for public health and global efforts to control the pandemic (Callaway, 2023). *Vaccine strategies:* The emergence of new variants underscored the importance of vaccination campaigns to achieve herd immunity with the possibility of booster shots and the development of updated vaccines targeting specific variants becoming routine (Tzenios et al., 2023). Vaccination campaigns were a critical component of the global response to COVID-19, to vaccinate large portions of the population to achieve herd immunity and reduce the spread of the virus (Lee & Haupt, 2021). While the specifics of these campaigns varied by country and region, there were common elements and steps involved in how COVID-19 vaccination campaigns worked (He et al., 2022). *Vaccine development and approval:* The process began with the development and clinical testing of COVID-19 vaccines by pharmaceutical companies and research institutions. Regulatory agencies like the US Food and Drug Administration (FDA) and the European Medicines Agency (EMA) reviewed the safety and efficacy data to approve vaccines for emergency or regular use (Kumar et al., 2023). *Vaccine distribution:* Once vaccines were approved, governments and health organizations worked on procuring and distributing vaccines, through partnerships with vaccine manufacturers and logistics providers to ensure equitable distribution (Kumar et al., 2023; Sparke & Levy, 2022).

Priority groups: To manage limited vaccine supplies, countries typically prioritized certain groups for vaccination, such as healthcare workers, older adults, and individuals with underlying health conditions. These priorities were often determined based on the risk of severe illness and death (Silliman Cohen & Bosk, 2020). *Vaccination sites:* Vaccination sites were set up in various locations, including hospitals, clinics, pharmacies, community centers, and mass vaccination sites. Mobile vaccination units were also used to reach underserved populations (He et al., 2022). *Appointment scheduling:* Many vaccination campaigns use appointment systems to manage the flow of people and minimize wait times. Online platforms or phone hotlines were often used for scheduling. (Charitos et al., 2022). *Vaccination process:* Individuals arriving at vaccination sites were registered, screened for eligibility, and provided with information about the vaccine. The vaccine was administered by trained healthcare professionals, usually as an intramuscular injection (He et al., 2022). *Monitoring and observation:* After receiving the vaccine, individuals were often observed for a brief period to monitor for any immediate adverse reactions (Charitos et al., 2022).

Vaccination cards and records: Individuals received documentation, such as vaccination cards, to verify their vaccination status. Some countries also established digital vaccine certificates or passports (He et al., 2022). *Second doses:* Many COVID-19 vaccines require two doses for full vaccination. Systems were set up to ensure individuals received their second doses within the recommended timeframe (Charitos et al., 2022). *Vaccine education and outreach programs:* Public health campaigns were launched to educate the public about the safety and efficacy of vaccines, address concerns, and encourage vaccine uptake (He et al., 2022). *Monitoring vaccine safety:* Continuous monitoring of vaccine safety was conducted through systems like the Vaccine Adverse Event Reporting System (VAERS) in the United States. Any adverse events were investigated, and appropriate actions were taken (Charitos et al., 2022). *Scaling up:* As vaccine supply increased, eligibility expanded to include more segments of the population. Mass vaccination events and outreach efforts were intensified (He et al., 2022). *Global vaccine distribution:* International efforts, such as COVAX, aimed to provide vaccines to low- and middle-income countries to ensure global access to vaccines (Charitos et al., 2022). *Booster shots:* Some countries introduced booster shots to enhance immunity and address waning vaccine effectiveness, especially against emerging variants of the virus (Shah & Coiado, 2023).

4.4 Conclusion

It's important to note that the success of vaccination campaigns depends on factors like vaccine supply, public trust, and logistical capabilities. These campaigns evolved over time as new variants of the virus emerged and as vaccination efforts continued to adapt to the changing situation. Public health authorities worked to overcome vaccine hesitancy and barriers to access to ensure as many people as possible were vaccinated to bring an end to the pandemic. Global collaboration by the scientific community to monitor and share data about the spread of the virus, and to coordinate their responses to new variants and strains played an important role in slowing down the further spread of COVID-19 around the world. These efforts were further supplemented by the adoption of strict measures by the governments and healthcare systems, including wearing masks, social distancing, and lockdowns, in response to the changing dynamics of subsequent waves and variant prevalence. Public education through effective communication was also vital to inform the public about the risks associated with new variants and the importance of vaccination and preventive measures.

4.5 Future lessons for managers

In this section, we provide some general lessons that managers might draw from how the subsequent waves of COVID-19 were handled. First and foremost, managers should understand and emphasize the importance of adaptability and flexibility in the face of uncertainty. The experience during the subsequent stages of the pandemic highlighted the importance of expecting the unexpected and the ability to pivot quickly in response to changing circumstances. Similarly, the later waves of the pandemic underlined the need to develop robust remote work policies and infrastructure, which managers may need to further refine to enhance their remote work capabilities and to ensure that their teams can continue to function effectively in challenging work environments. In this context, managers would need to prioritize the well-being and mental health of their employees and be proactive in offering support and resources due to the unique challenges faced by them during times of crisis. At the same time, it is vital to have clear, transparent, and timely communication and this would require managers to refine their communication strategies to keep employees informed, engaged, and aligned with organizational goals during a crisis such as the COVID-19 pandemic.

Managers should also lead their organizations to invest in robust crisis planning and preparedness, which may include contingency plans for various scenarios to ensure the availability and optimal utilization of essential resources and regular updating of plans based on lessons learned from previous experiences. In this process, the use of emerging technologies would be very critical to enable business continuity as underscored by the pandemic. Managers should continue to invest in and leverage technology to streamline their processes, enhance collaboration, and facilitate remote work. On a related note, the interconnected nature of the world became even more apparent during the pandemic. Managers should understand that challenges in one part of the world can have ripple effects globally and they should encourage global collaboration for information sharing and problem-solving accordingly.

The subsequent waves of the pandemic continued to wreak havoc on the economy, especially causing disruptions in supply chains, which emphasized the need to build resilient supply chain networks. Managers should assess and strengthen the resilience of their existing supply chains and develop more resilient supply chains and logistics systems to mitigate risks. Similarly, scenario planning should be a regular part of strategic management. Managers need to anticipate potential future disruptions, consider various scenarios, and develop plans to navigate through them. At the same time, organizations should continue to invest in health and safety measures to protect employees, including the provision of necessary resources, training, and protocols to ensure a safe working environment. Finally, it is crucial for managers to conduct periodic reviews of how different aspects of their businesses and organizations are managed during periods of crisis. Identifying both successes and failures during these experiences would provide valuable insights to managers for future crisis management.

5   COVID-19 differences in national responses

Different strokes

5.1   National difference in COVID-19 responses

COVID-19, an unprecedented global crisis, unveiled a complex web of national responses that highlighted the intricate interplay of politics, healthcare systems, socio-economic factors, and cultural norms. This essay delves into the differences in national responses to COVID-19, showcasing the diverse strategies employed by governments worldwide. From the outset, nations exhibited a range of responses to the pandemic. Some embraced aggressive containment measures, while others adopted more lenient approaches, reflecting unique contexts and priorities. Countries like New Zealand and Australia swiftly implemented strict lockdowns, aiming to eliminate the virus from their borders. These nations prioritized public health over short-term economic concerns, and their efforts resulted in effective virus containment. Some countries, like Sweden, initially adopted a more relaxed approach, emphasizing individual responsibility and avoiding widespread lockdowns. This approach sought to balance public health with minimizing economic disruptions, although it generated significant debate and controversy. By contrast, nations like China used their centralized governance structures to implement very strict measures, including mass quarantines and surveillance with forced restrictions on travel and social interactions (Liu et al., 2021).

While these measures effectively curtailed the virus's spread, concerns were raised about civil liberties. Countries with robust healthcare systems, such as Germany and South Korea, leveraged comprehensive testing, contact tracing, and public communication. Their adaptable strategies mitigated the virus's impact while maintaining socio-economic stability. Nations with limited healthcare infrastructure, like many in Africa, faced challenges in responding effectively. They grappled with insufficient testing capabilities, medical resources, and the need to balance public health with economic imperatives.

Recent studies identify significant differences in the countries' responses to COVID-19 (Leung et al., 2020; Sharma et al., 2020), with some acting quickly with strict measures, such as lockdowns and border closures, to successfully contain its initial spread, and thus minimize the number of cases and deaths (e.g., Australia, New Zealand, Taiwan, and Vietnam) but others have

DOI: 10.4324/9781003227113-6

not been as proactive and have suffered more as a result (e.g., Italy, Spain, UK, and USA). Interestingly, some countries have faltered after their initial success with very strict measures (e.g., India, South Korea, and Singapore), while others have allowed COVID-19 to spread almost unchecked (e.g., Brazil and Russia). Similarly, organizations in different countries are also coping with COVID-19 in diverse ways (Brueck, 2020), such as using open-source and collaborative responses to produce medical equipment and supplies, develop and test vaccines, and track the spread of the virus across communities (Chesbrough, 2020). Some organizations have also responded more quickly than others, by adopting new ways to run their operations, such as allowing their employees to work from home (Dingel & Neiman, 2020), and schools and universities switching to online teaching (Crawford et al., 2020).

Similar differences are being observed in the way people, both individuals and social groups such as families, friends, and colleagues, are responding to COVID-19 crisis. For example, people in collectivistic cultures that emphasize the importance of close relations with other community members (e.g., China, Japan, and South Korea) have responded with prompt community responses and volunteering efforts, which have made dealing with a strict measure like lockdowns relatively easier, and helped maintain social harmony during these challenging times (De Vries, 2020). By contrast, people in individualistic cultures that focus on taking individual responsibility and looking out for oneself more than others (e.g., Australia, UK, and USA) have seen selfish behaviors, such as panic buying in supermarkets, people not wearing masks in public places, and protestors gathering despite the huge risk of catching the coronavirus infection (Rathod et al., 2020).

National responses were shaped by a myriad of factors, including differences in the institutions and systems used by different countries to manage the pandemic. *Governance systems:* Political systems influenced responses, with democracies focusing on public consensus and authoritarian regimes imposing top-down measures (Liu et al., 2021). *Healthcare systems:* Countries with robust healthcare systems could better manage cases, while others faced capacity constraints. *Socio-economic status:* Economic considerations influenced approaches, as some nations weighed lockdowns against economic stability. *Cultural norms:* Societal behaviors and cultural norms played a role in shaping responses, and influencing compliance with preventive measures. *Public trust:* Effective communication bolstered public trust, encouraging compliance, while misinformation eroded trust and hindered responses. These differences in national responses yielded both lessons and challenges. For example, diverse approaches provided a rich spectrum of strategies for managing future pandemics. Successes, such as New Zealand's elimination strategy, underscore the importance of swift, science-based responses. On the other hand, variations in responses also underscore the need for international collaboration and information sharing to combat global threats effectively.

Past research shows that effective management of global crises needs a comprehensive approach that focuses on their impact across a diverse range of issues, including economic, environmental, healthcare, political, social, and other areas (Victor & Ahmed, 2019). In this context, culture is recognized as a major factor that drives the differences in the response to such disasters, including the willingness to accept the challenges and adopt the advice from the experts to be able to control the severity of their impact (Knipsel, 2020; Stann, 2020). However, many of these simply describe the differences in the national responses to these crises without any theoretical explanations (e.g., De Vries, 2020; De Witte, 2020; Knipsel, 2020; Rathod et al., 2020; Stann, 2020). Others focus on the impact of customs and traditional beliefs (Agusto et al., 2015), socio-cultural practices (Adongo et al., 2016), community beliefs and fears (Grimaud & Legagneur, 2011), and traditional religious practices (Manguvo & Mafuvadze, 2015), despite growing evidence about the importance of cultural diversity in managing health outcomes (Ancarani et al., 2016). Therefore, despite their useful insights about cultural differences in the responses to public health crises, there is no comprehensive conceptual framework based on strong theoretical foundations to provide guidance to public health managers, policy makers, and academic researchers (Wursten, 2020).

We address this important research gap by exploring the impact of national cultural values on the process that has driven the national responses to COVID-19, in terms of their level of readiness to handle such a large-scale healthcare crisis and prevent its negative outcomes. We begin with a review of the literature on the differences in the national responses to major virus outbreaks (including COVID-19) and national cultural frameworks (e.g., Hofstede, 1980, 1991, 2001; Minkov, 2018). Next, we combine Hofstede's (2001) framework with institutional theory to develop our conceptual model with specific hypotheses on the impact of four relevant national cultural values, namely power distance (PDI), individualism (IDV), long-term orientation (LTO), and uncertainty avoidance (UAI) on COVID-19 outcomes, such as number of deaths (DEATHS) and recoveries (RECOVER) as a ratio to the total COVID-19 cases diagnosed so far. We also investigate the mediating role played by key socio-economic indicators, such as per capita gross domestic product (GDPC), human development index (HDI), income inequality Index (GINI), and public health expenditure (HEX) as a ratio of GDP, and public healthcare infrastructure in terms of per capita number of hospital beds (BEDS), physicians (PHYS), and COVID-19 tests (TESTS) in this process.

Using secondary data published by reliable sources (e.g., World Bank, WHO, and UNDP), we find support for the impact of four national cultural values (PDI, IDV, LTO, and UAI) on three socio-economic indicators (GDPC, HDI, GINI, and HEX), three public health infrastructure (BEDS, PHYS, and TESTS) and two COVID-19 outcomes (DEATHS and RECOVER). Overall, we find that national culture has an impact on the macro-level socio-economic performance and public health infrastructure but this may not be enough to deliver positive public health outcomes in the absence of effective decision-making by public health officials and government leaders, especially during a global health crisis. We discuss the conceptual contribution and practical implications of our findings along with some limitations of our methodology and directions for future research.

5.2   Cultural differences in COVID-19 responses

Given its global spread and devastating socio-economic impact, addressing and managing COVID-19 require concerted efforts at many levels, including public policy and governance at the institutional level but probably more importantly, implementation at the community and individual levels, to avoid any long-term damage to our efforts to improve social equality, inclusion, and personal well-being as well as reduce discrimination (United Nations, 2020). In this context, the role of national culture and institutions could be extremely important as any efforts to respond to the socio-economic challenges posed by COVID-19 would be conditioned by the national cultural values and need to be implemented mainly by the public institutions in collaboration with the private sector and individual citizens (Kurdin, 2020). In this context, recent reports demonstrate significant differences in the way people are responding to the tough measures announced by their governments (e.g., De Vries, 2020).

For example, Japan was initially quite successful in its fight against COVID-19 because of the collective action of the Japanese people, "Japan has succeeded in countering both the initial advance of COVID-19 and a complacency spike. Reasons proffered have been many and varied. One that may yet attract increasing attention is its culture of collectivism" (De Vries, 2020). In contrast, many Americans were protesting against preventive measures like social distancing, calling these against fundamental principles of "independence", "liberty", and "free will", which are highly valued in individualistic societies such as the United States (De Vries, 2020). Unfortunately, such actions hampered the collective response to fight against COVID-19. Similarly, the effectiveness and necessity of wearing facemasks to slow down the spread of the virus in the community have also generated very different responses around the world. For example, there have been significant public expressions and protests against wearing facemasks as a way to highlight individual freedom of choice in Western countries characterized by their individualistic cultures but it has been much more socially acceptable in Asian countries with relatively more collectivistic cultures (Leung, 2020).

Past research on the role of culture in managing global disasters such as pandemics also documents significant differences in the willingness of political leaders and heads of public institutions, to acknowledge the severity and enormity of the challenges and accept the advice from the experts, in order to be able to control their impact in an effective manner (Knipsel, 2020; Stann, 2020). However, most of these studies are either descriptive with no theoretical foundations (e.g., De Vries, 2020; De Witte, 2020; Knipsel, 2020; Rathod et al., 2020; Stann, 2020) or focus on the unique aspects of different cultures, such as community beliefs and fears (Grimaud & Legagneur,

2011), traditional religious practices (Manguvo & Mafuvadze, 2015), customs and beliefs (Agusto et al., 2015), and socio-cultural practices (Adongo et al., 2016), despite the importance of cultural diversity in managing health outcomes (Ancarani et al., 2016). Hence, there is still no comprehensive conceptual framework to guide public policy makers, political leaders and officials, and academic researchers (Wursten, 2020). We address this gap by combining Hofstede's national cultural framework with institutional theory to study the differences in the national responses to COVID-19.

5.3 National cultural values

Societal culture is generally conceptualized as "a system of shared values, beliefs, and behavioral norms, which are learned and passed from one generation to the next through the laws, policies, and actions of a society" (Pacheco et al., 2016, p. 607). According to Hofstede (1980; 1991; 2001), culture is akin to mental software, which is quite stable in nature and responsible for people in a particular society to be 'programmed' to think and act in a similar manner. This view is based on the argument that the shared social norms and cultural values have shaped the socio-political institutions in every country, which in turn influence the policies and procedures adopted by their organizations and the responses of the employees to the same (Hofstede, 2001; Hofstede et al., 2010; Smith et al., 1996). In this context, more studies focus on the IDV-collectivism dimension (e.g., Stavrou & Kilaniotis, 2010; Thompson & Phua, 2005) compared to Hofstede's (2001) other national cultural values, including PDI, masculinity-femininity, UAI, and LTO (Wong & Cheng, 2020).

Past research shows a significant impact of national culture on organizational structures, leadership behaviors, negotiation processes, and human resource management policies, with useful implications for career development, training design, and multicultural management in general (Smith, 1992). Recent studies explore the impact of culture on employee attitudes and outcomes, such as participative leadership (Miao et al., 2013), empowerment (Fong & Snape, 2015), job satisfaction (Pacheco et al., 2016), organizational policies, such as flexible and remote working arrangements (Peretz et al., 2018), and organizational culture (Cunha et al., 2019). For example, Miao et al. (2013) argue that Western-style management practices that encourage employee participation may not be successful in high PDI cultures (e.g., China) due to their authoritarian styles of leadership with top-down decision-making approach. Cunha et al. (2019) confirm this by showing that efforts to change the organizational culture to one that encourages employees to "speak up" can lead to "tensions and contradictions" and reveal organizational paradoxes, especially if such a cultural change is in conflict with the prevailing national culture (e.g., high PDI).

Pacheco et al. (2016) use four waves of the European Values Study with a sample of 13 countries to show a stable influence of traditional societal values on job satisfaction during 1981–2008 period. More recently, Peretz et al. (2018) used GLOBE national cultural values with a sample of 21 countries to show that organizations in the countries with high IDV, low PDI, low UAI, high future orientation, high assertiveness, high gender egalitarianism, high humane orientation, and high-performance orientation, have a higher preference for flexible working arrangement (LaBerge et al., 2020). However, despite their useful contributions, most of these studies are restricted to a relatively smaller group of countries and they do not consider the impact of broader national-level socio-economic indicators and public institutional infrastructure, hence their impact on public services outcomes is still not clear, which could be particularly important during a global crisis. We address this research gap by investigating the impact of national cultural values on how effectively various countries have handled the ongoing COVID-19.

5.4   Institutional perspective

Institutional theory is a theoretical perspective that drives the impact of country-level contextual factors (e.g., national cultural values) on the relationships between organizational actions and their outcomes (North, 1991). Institutions put constraints on how different social, economic, and political entities interact with each other; consisting of both informal (e.g., customs, codes of conduct, sanctions, taboos, and traditions) as well as formal (e.g., constitutions, laws, property rights, rules, and regulations) constraints (North, 1991). Institutions help create and maintain order by reducing uncertainty and building trust in exchanges that involve two or more entities. Institutions evolve with time and act as bridges between the past and the present with the future to explain how cultures and economies grow, stagnate, or decline (North, 1991). Institutional theory suggests that although organization structure enables action, it also puts constraints on how organizations respond to change and crisis, which can be explained with a culture-practice fit perspective (Minbaeva et al., 2018).

North (1991) argues that any country's ability to implement new rules and regulations depends on the prevailing national cultural values and the awareness levels of its citizens. In the context of the ongoing COVID-19 or any other global crisis, it means that the success of any government actions or directives would depend on the effectiveness of public institutions and the extent to which people are willing to abide by any new regulations. For example, countries with capable governments with decisive political leaders (e.g., Jacinda Ardern in New Zealand) have been able to communicate effectively with the public in a factual and transparent manner that has helped them not only build their trust and confidence but also elicit positive actions and compliance with the harsh measures, including lockdowns, social distancing and quarantines (Wittenberg-Cox, 2020). Similarly, governments that developed their strategies based on the available facts and implemented them quickly (e.g., Taiwan) were able to save numerous lives due to their timely action, which again earned them the respect and loyalty of their citizens and helped them avoid the disastrous economic and public health outcomes suffered by other countries that delayed their actions (e.g., UK and USA). Finally, many leaders (e.g., Justin Trudeau in Canada) communicated directly and frequently with the media and the public to convey their empathy for the loss and suffering experienced by their people, which resulted in a more effective handling of the situation.

5.5 National cultural values

5.5.1 PDI

PDI represents the extent to which the less powerful members of a society expect and accept unequal distribution of power (Hofstede, 2001). As a result, less powerful members of high PDI societies tend to tolerate the imbalances in power and are afraid to disagree with those in powerful positions, such as politicians, business and community leaders, etc. (Miao et al., 2013). In contrast, those with higher powers exercise their powers to accumulate social privileges and economic wealth (Hofstede, 2001). Hence, it is not surprising to see managers in high PDI cultures abuse their powers and exploit their subordinates, which often goes unchallenged by the employees in lower-level positions due to their perceived lack of power (Cunha et al., 2019). High PDI cultures also suffer from greater information asymmetry between people with different levels of power because of the inherent social inequality in such cultures (Jain & Jain, 2018). This information asymmetry may result in a lack of transparency and information sharing with those at lower levels of the social hierarchy (Cunha et al., 2019), which could have disastrous outcomes during a global health crisis by not allowing those with lower levels of power to take the appropriate actions to save their health (Bryant et al., 2007).

Past research shows that PDI has a negative association with economic (Tang & Koveos, 2008) and human development (Matusitz & Musambira, 2013) in general, and with GDP (Cox et al., 2011) and HDI (Scholl & Schermuly, 2020). In high PDI cultures, people with more power do not allow those below them to earn higher incomes and become more prosperous to maintain the PDI, which results in high-income inequality (Hofstede, 2001). This high-income inequality impedes socio-economic development by preventing a fair distribution of resources such as education, employment, healthcare, and housing, which can only be improved by legislative actions (e.g., tax and welfare policies), entrepreneurial activities, and technological changes according to the institutional perspective (Tang & Koveos, 2008). Borisova et al. (2017) also find a negative link between PDI and public health perceptions because high PDI cultures tend to be more autocratic and hierarchical, which may result in making their public health systems inefficient and not allowing their benefits to reach the lower sections of the society. Based on this discussion, we expect PDI to relate negatively with (a) per capita GDP, (b) HDI, (c) per capita public HEX, and positively with (d) GINI.

5.5.2   IDV-Collectivism

IDV represents the extent to which people take personal responsibility for their actions and focus on individual achievements, with a high degree of self-orientation; whereas, collectivism represents the extent to which people take collective responsibility and are socialized into cohesive in-groups, with group goals and norms guiding their behavior more than personal goals and ambition (Hofstede, 2001). Individualistic traits include assertiveness, competitiveness, initiative, and self-assurance; while collectivistic traits include conformity, dependence, empathy, self-control, and self-sacrifice (Church, 2000). Past research uses the institutional perspective to show a positive association between IDV and socio-economic indicators because individualistic cultures emphasize the importance of private enterprise and risk-taking behaviors that are required for economic growth and human development (e.g., Cox et al., 2011; Scholl & Schermuly, 2020). Moreover, the impersonal and goal-oriented achievement standards coupled with a lower need to conform to societal norms, associated with individualistic entrepreneurs, also help them grow their businesses by tackling competition and garnering more resources for themselves (Tang & Koveos, 2008). Similarly, people in individualistic cultures also rate their national health system more favorably because they expect to be taken care of by virtue of being an individual worthy of being provided the best service by the institutions funded by their tax dollars (Borisova et al., 2017). Hence, we expect IDV to relate positively with (a) per capita GDP, (b) HDI, (c) per capita public HEX, and negatively with (d) GINI.

5.5.3   LTO

LTO represents a focus on the future, characterized by personal traits such as perseverance, prudence, thrift, and a sense of responsibility, which drive people to behave in a respectable manner by fulfilling their obligations mandated by social relationships (Hofstede, 2001). In contrast, short-term orientation is associated with a focus on the present, which results in respect for tradition, stability, and avoidance of risk to prevent losing "face" in front of significant others. Cultures with higher LTO have higher rates of individual and household savings, which may help people in these cultures prevent socio-economic disasters by having sufficient protection in case of job loss or sickness (Tang & Koveos, 2008). Although improved financial markets and availability of consumer credit may reduce the need for precautionary savings, the higher costs of living (particularly healthcare and elderly care) may require people to save more for their retirement.

In this context, past research uses the institutional perspective to show a positive association between LTO and socio-economic indicators because governments in such cultures are more likely to invest in their future in terms of education, healthcare, and other public infrastructure, which are essential for further economic growth and human development (e.g., Cox et al., 2011; Scholl & Schermuly, 2020). However, there is no evidence that LTO may affect public HEX that would create positive outcomes despite its importance for ensuring the overall objective and subjective well-being of the people in any society. Accordingly, we expect LTO to relate positively with (a) per capita GDP, (b) HDI, (c) per capita public HEX, and negatively with (d) GINI.

5.5.4 UAI

UAI represents the extent to which people feel uncomfortable with uncertain, unknown, or unstructured situations (Hofstede, 2001); hence, people in countries with high UAI tend to be more conservative and risk-averse. Cultures with high UAI also follow strict behavioral codes, laws, and rules, with limited information sharing (Hofstede, 2001). People in such cultures also have lower tolerance for ambiguity and uncertainty with a high need for structure and organization compared to those in low UAI cultures. Hofstede (1980) identifies three components of UAI, including rule orientation, employment stability, and stress, which influence people in less developed economies to a greater extent due to the instability of employment and stressful work environment (Tang & Koveos, 2008).

Past research shows a negative association between UAI and socio-economic indicators because people in such cultures tend to avoid taking risks, which may prevent them from realizing their true potential in terms of economic growth and human development (e.g., Cox et al., 2011; Scholl & Schermuly, 2020). There is also a general consensus based on the institutional perspective about the positive association between the objective and subjective indicators of socio-economic development and the level of industrialization and modernization, which makes most people in developed countries experience higher levels of subjective well-being than those in the less developed countries (Tang & Koveos, 2008). However, there is no significant link between UAI and evaluation of public health systems by people in such cultures despite the importance of having efficient healthcare to reduce the uncertainty and risk in their everyday lives (Borisova et al., 2017). Based on these results, we expect UAI to relate negatively with (a) per capita GDP, (b) HDI, (c) per capita public HEX, and positively with (d) GINI.

5.6 Social-economic indicators

GDP has been a popular indicator of the economic performance of countries for almost a century and it remains popular despite the emergence of other indicators, such as Measure of Economic Welfare (MEW) or Gross National

Happiness (GNH), which aim to measure overall well-being and not just the economic performance (Monni & Spaventa, 2013; Natoli & Zuhair, 2011). HDI is another measure that taps into the overall level of development of a country in terms of being able to take care of the welfare of its citizens (Kalimeris et al., 2020). Past research also uses public HEX as an indicator of the quality of public health albeit with mixed evidence about its impact on improving public health outcomes (Self & Grabowski, 2003). Overall, there is considerable consensus on the usefulness of these socio-economic indicators in evaluating the general health of the economy of a country and the well-being of its people. Therefore, in this chapter, we combine Hofstede's national cultural framework with the institutional perspective, to include per capita GDP, HDI, and per capita public HEX as important variables in the process by which national cultural values may influence public health infrastructure and its outcomes in the COVID-19 context.

5.7   Public health infrastructure

Past research provides mixed evidence about the association between GDP and public HEX. Rana et al. (2020) address this using panel data for 161 countries during 1995–2014 period to show that economic growth can only explain about 43% of the variance in global public HEX growth and that income shocks have a stronger influence on the HEX of high (vs. low) income countries. However, past research also finds no significant influence of national culture on public health outcomes, such as life expectancy, maternal and infant mortality rates, etc. because the impact of national culture on individuals' decisions about their health may be dominated by other factors such as environmental conditions (e.g., weather) that may affect the spread of disease (Gamlath, 2017). Similarly, rapid urbanization may lead to adverse health outcomes due to easier spread of infectious diseases such as cholera, flu, and typhoid fever (Gamlath, 2017).

Interestingly, the above view ignores the likely impact of poor decision-making by public health officials and political leaders in the face of a global health crisis as seen in the case of ongoing COVID-19 (Patterson, 2020; Qato, 2020). In this context, past research shows a positive link between public HEX and its outcomes, such as infant mortality and life expectancy rates (Kim & Lane, 2013). We use the institutional perspective to examine the indirect influence of national cultural values on COVID-19 outcomes through socio-economic indicators and public health infrastructure. Specifically, we posit that socio-economic indicators such as GDPC, HDI, and HEX would have positive effects on public health infrastructure (e.g., per capita number of BEDS, PHYS, and TESTS available to diagnose the patients). Hence, we expect GDPC, HDI, and HEX to relate positively with each other and negatively with GINI. We also expect HDI and HEX to relate positively and GINI to relate negatively with per capita numbers of (a) BEDS, (b) PHYS, and (c) TESTS.

5.8   Public health outcomes

Past research shows a positive association between public HEX and public health outcomes, such as lower infant mortality rate and higher life expectancy at birth (Kim & Lane, 2013). However, others reveal relatively poorer public health outcomes such as higher infant mortality and obesity coupled with lower life expectancy and overall well-being in high-income countries (e.g., USA) despite much higher per capita expenditure on health than others, mostly due to poor education, alcohol consumption, and tobacco use (Oney, 2012). More recently, Krieger (2019) shows that the quality of public policy has a significant impact on the health outcomes of poor people. Accordingly, we expect public health infrastructure (e.g., per capita number of BEDS and PHYS) to lead to positive COVID-19 outcomes, such as a lower number of deaths and a higher number of recoveries.

5.9   Methodology

We used secondary data analysis with publicly reported indicators from reliable sources (e.g., World Bank, WHO, and UNDP) to operationalize all the constructs and test our hypotheses. Specifically, we used national cultural values scores from Hofstede (2001), socio-economic (GDPC and HDI) and public health (HEX, BEDS, and PHYS) indicators from the year 2018, and all the public health outcomes related to COVID-19 were as on 21 August 2021. This temporal separation between the independent and dependent variables helps us eliminate concerns about common method bias, endogeneity, and reverse causality (Mertens et al., 2017). All our measures are also either indices or ratios, which helps avoid confounding effects of any between-country differences (e.g., total population or total number of COVID-19 cases). Table 5.1 shows the sample profile using three levels for each characteristic with the total number of countries for each characteristic being subject to the availability of data for that characteristic (Figure 5.1).

- *National cultural values* (PDI, IDV, LTO, and UAI). Country scores for each of these national cultural dimensions (Hofstede et al., 2010)
- GDPC. GDP for each country (in million US dollars) divided by its population in millions for the year 2018 (World Bank, 2020).
- HDI. A composite index ranking countries in terms of human development based on three dimensions, namely life expectancy index, education index, and income index, for the year 2018 (UNDP, 2020).
- GINI. A measure of the distribution of income across a population, ranging from 0 = perfect equality to 1 = perfect inequality (UNDP, 2020).
- *Public* HEX. Current expenditure on public health by a country as a percentage of its GDP for the year 2018 (UNDP, 2020).
- *Public health infrastructure*. Number of BEDS and PHYS for the year 2018 (UNDP, 2020), and number of TESTS as of 21 August 2021 (Worldometer, 2020).

Table 5.1 Sample profile (N = 212)

Sample characteristics	No. of countries	% age	Sample characteristics	No. of countries	% age
PDI			IDV		
11–46	23	32.9%	6–27	24	34.8%
47–68	24	34.3%	28–59	22	31.9%
69–104	23	32.9%	60–91	23	33.3%
LTO			UAI		
4–31	30	33.7%	8–58	22	31.9%
32–60	30	33.7%	59–82	23	33.3%
61–100	29	32.6%	83–112	24	34.8%
GDPC in US$			HDI		
660–7393	55	32.5%	0.38–0.66	56	32.2%
7509–21075	57	33.7%	0.67–0.80	60	34.5%
22674–112532	57	33.7%	0.81–0.95	58	33.3%
GINI			Per Capita Public HEX in US$		
660–7393	55	32.5%	8.65–148.78	57	33.5%
7509–21075	57	33.7%	159.48–869.08	57	33.5%
22674–112532	57	33.7%	902.14–10246.14	56	32.9%
BEDS per thousand population			PHYS per thousand population		
0.1–1.40	57	31.7%	0.02–0.82	62	34.1%
1.50–3.40	62	34.4%	0.84–2.37	60	33.0%
3.50–14.35	61	33.9%	2.39–8.19	60	33.0%
TESTS per thousand population			COVID-19 deaths to total cases ratio (DEATHS)		
0.00–162.57	71	33.5%	0.00–0.01	77	36.3%
162.57–781.43	71	33.5%	0.01–0.02	65	30.7%
781.43–13679.77	70	33.0%	0.02–0.19	70	33.0%
COVID-19 recoveries to total cases ratio (RECOVER)					
0.00–0.87	71	33.5%			
0.87–0.95	71	33.5%			
0.95–1.00	70	33.0%			

Note: The total number of countries for each characteristic is subject to availability of data.

- *COVID-19 outcomes.* Two indicators, namely number of deaths due to COVID-19 as a percentage of total cases (DEATHS), and a number of recoveries as a percentage of total COVID-19 cases (RECOVER) as of 21 August 2021 (Worldometer, 2020).
- *Control variables.* Three demographic indicators reported by UNDP (2020), including the percentage of population above the age of 65 years (POP65), urban population as the percentage of total population living in urban areas (URBAN), and population density per square kilometer (PDEN), due to their impact on COVID-19 outcomes (Leung et al., 2020)

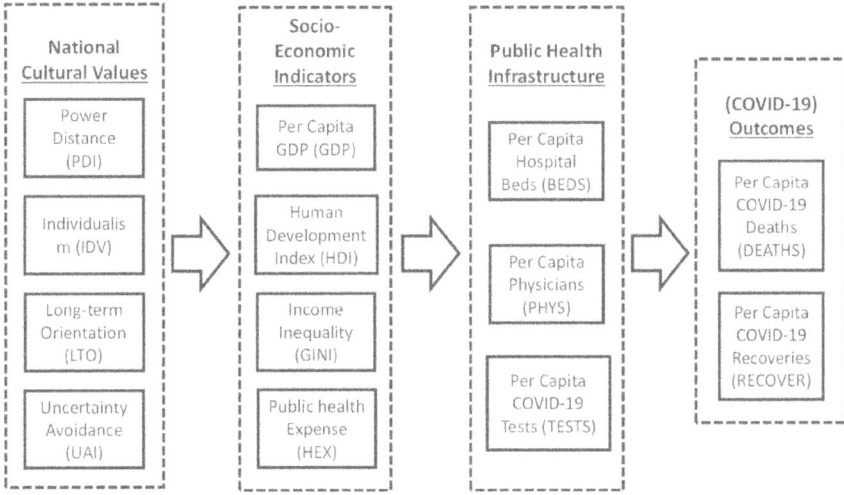

Figure 5.1 Shows our conceptual framework with all the expected relationships.

5.10   Data analysis and results

We use path analysis with SmartPLS 3.3 to test all the expected relationships because we have a relatively small sample (N = 212) with many ratios and indices in our data that may not be normally distributed, and because our conceptual model is quite complex with many constructs and relationships (Hair et al., 2019). All the VIF (Variance Inflation Factor) values are less than the recommended cut-off value of three, thus multi-collinearity is not a concern (Hair et al., 2019). Next, the average R-square value for all the variables is .44 with all the individual values higher than .20 (GDPC = .38, HDI = .55, GINI = .61, HEX = .81, BEDS = .51, PHYS = .71, TESTS = .21, DEATHS = .29, RECOVER = .26), hence the model explains a significant proportion of variance in these variables. High values of blindfolding-based cross-validated redundancy measure Q^2 for all the variables (.27–.74) also confirm the predictive accuracy of the partial least squares (PLS) path model (Hair et al., 2019). Finally, a low standardized root mean squared residual (SRMR) (.048) and high normed fit index (NFI) (.90) also show a good model-fit. Table 5.2 shows the correlations and descriptive statistics for all the variables and Table 5.3 reports the results of the path analysis.

First, PDI has significant negative associations with GDPC (β = −.42, p < .001) and HEX (β = −.15, p < .01) but not with HDI (β = −.03, p > .05) and GINI (β = .02, p > .05). However, IDV has significant positive associations with GDPC (β = .27, p < .01), HEX (β = .19, p < .05), HDI (β = .15, p < .05), and negative with GINI (β = −.25, p < .05). Next, LTO has significant positive associations with GDPC (β = .28, p < .001), HDI (β = .17, p < .05), and HEX (β = .15, p < .05) but not with GINI (β = −.09, p > .05).

Table 5.2 Correlations and descriptive statistics

Variables	1	2	3	4	5	6	7	8	9	10	11	12
1 PDI	1.00											
2 IDV	-.65	1.00										
3 LTO	.00	.08	1.00									
4 UAI	.26	-.22	-.02	1.00								
5 Per Capita GDP in US$ (GDPC)	-.45	.46	.21	-.09	1.00							
6 HDI	-.33	.42	.29	-.02	.69	1.00						
7 GINI	.35	-.40	-.33	-.02	-.63	-.81	1.00					
8 Per Capita Public HEX	-.60	.63	.20	-.09	.73	.60	-.59	1.00				
9 TESTS per million population (TESTS)	-.52	.41	.12	-.27	.29	.26	-.33	.31	1.00			
10 Hospital beds per thousand population (BEDS)	-.23	.32	.48	.28	.31	.50	-.61	.31	.21	1.00		
11 PHYS per thousand population	-.49	.55	.27	.11	.56	.73	-.78	.61	.27	.58	1.00	
12 COVID-19 deaths as % of total cases (DEATHS)	.23	-.24	-.05	.15	-.10	-.04	.06	-.04	-.21	-.11	-.04	1.00
13 COVID-19 recoveries as % of total cases (RECOVER)	.06	-.02	.14	.12	.06	.05	-.04	.10	.13	.06	.11	-.02
Mean	58.47	43.60	68.03	46.19	19830.71	0.72	19.08	1149.67	949.40	3.15	1.83	0.02
Standard deviation	21.16	23.99	23.62	23.33	19831.54	0.15	9.98	1845.56	1733.99	2.75	1.55	0.02

$^*p < .05$; $^{**}p < .01$

Table 5.3 Path analysis (SmartPLS 3.0) output

Hypothesized relationships	β	Result
PDI → Per capita GDP	−.42***	Supported
PDI → HDI	−.03	Not supported
PDI → Public HEX	−.15*	Supported
PDI → GINI	.02	Not supported
IDV → Per capita GDP	.27**	Supported
IDV → HDI	.19*	Supported
IDV → Public HEX	.15*	Supported
IDV → GINI	−.25**	Supported
LTO → Per capita GDP	.28**	Supported
LTO → HDI	.17*	Supported
LTO → Public HEX	.15*	Supported
LTO → GINI	−.09	Not supported
UAI → Per capita GDP	−.18*	Supported
UAI → HDI	−.19*	Supported
UAI → Public HEX	.02	Not supported
UAI → GINI	.24**	Supported
Per capita GDP → HDI	.59***	Supported
Per capita GDP → Public HEX	.74***	Supported
Per capita GDP → GINI	−.58***	Supported
HDI → BEDS/'000 pop	.03	Not supported
HDI → PHYS/'000 pop	.45***	Supported
HDI → TESTS/Million pop	.15*	Supported
GINI → BEDS/'000 pop	−.78***	Supported
GINI → PHYS/'000 pop	−.32**	Supported
GINI → TESTS/Million pop	−.05	Not supported
Public HEX → BEDS/'000 pop	.23**	Supported
Public HEX → PHYS/'000 pop	.26**	Supported
Public HEX → TESTS/Million pop	.54***	Supported
BEDS → COVID-19 deaths (% of total cases)	−.04	Not supported
BEDS → COVID-19 recoveries (% of total cases)	.27**	Supported
PHYS → COVID-19 deaths (% of total cases)	−.14*	Supported
PHYS → COVID-19 recoveries (% of total cases)	.19*	Supported

*β = Standardized β coefficient; * p < .05; ** p < .01; *** p < .001.*

Finally, UAI has a significant negative association with GDPC ($\beta = -.18$, $p < .05$) and HDI ($\beta = -.19$, $p > .05$) but no significant association with HEX ($\beta = .02$, $p > .05$) and a significant positive association with GINI ($\beta = .24$, $p < .01$).

Next, GDPC has significant positive associations with both HDI ($\beta = .59$, $p < .001$), HEX ($\beta = .74$, $p < .001$), and negative with GINI ($\beta = -.58$, $p < .001$). HDI has significant positive associations with PHYS ($\beta = .45$, $p < .001$) and TESTS ($\beta = .15$, $p < .05$) but not with BEDS ($\beta = .03$, $p > .05$). GINI has significant negative associations with BEDS ($\beta = -.78$, $p < .001$) and PHYS ($\beta = -.32$, $p < .01$) but not with TESTS ($\beta = -.05$, $p > .05$). HEX has significant positive associations with BEDS ($\beta = .23$, $p < .01$), PHYS ($\beta = .26$, $p < .01$), and TESTS ($\beta = .54$, $p < .001$). Next, BEDS has a significant positive association with RECOVER ($\beta = .27$, $p < .01$) but not with DEATHS

(β = $-.04$, p > .05). In contrast, PHYS has a significant negative association with DEATHS (β = $-.14$, p < .05) and a positive association with RECOVER (β = .19, p < .05). Finally, none of the three control variables have any significant association with the two COVID-19 outcomes. Specifically, POP65 has no significant association with either DEATHS (β = .04, p > .05) or RE-COVER (β = $-.04$, p > .05). Similarly, URBAN has no significant association with either DEATHS (β = .12, p > .05) or RECOVER (β = .06, p > .05). Finally, PDEN also has no significant association with either DEATHS (β = .02, p > .05) or RECOVER (β = .03, p > .05). Thus, demographic indicators such as aging population, urban population, and population density do not seem to directly affect COVID-19 outcomes.

5.11 Discussion and implications

This chapter introduces a multi-stage conceptual model to explain the differences in the national responses to the ongoing COVID-19 by exploring the impact of four national cultural values (PDI, IDV, LTO, and UAI) on four socio-economic indicators (GDPC, HDI, GINI, and HEX), public health infrastructure (BEDS, PHYS, and TESTS), and COVID-19 outcomes (DEATHS and RECOVER). We test all the expected relationships using secondary data from reliable sources (e.g., World Bank, WHO, Worldometer, and UNDP). Overall, we find evidence about the impact of four national cultural values on the four socio-economic indicators and their subsequent effects on the three public health infrastructure indicators and two COVID-19 outcomes. These findings suggest that although national culture may influence a country's socio-economic development and public health infrastructure, it may not be enough to deliver positive public health outcomes during a global health crisis, in the absence of effective decision-making by public health officials and leaders in national and local governments. Next, we discuss these findings and their implications in more detail.

Hofstede and Hofstede (2005) argue that while culture remains stable over time, rituals and practices (e.g., church attendance) are more susceptible to change. Past research shows that national cultural values have significant associations with economic (Tang & Koveos, 2008) and human development (Matusitz & Musambira, 2013) as reflected by socio-economic indicators, such as GDP (Cox et al., 2011) and HDI (Scholl & Schermuly, 2020). Researchers explain these findings by arguing that these national cultural values influence the way societies are organized and how people behave with each other and with public institutions in their countries. For example, Borisova et al. (2017) find a significant association between national cultural values and perceptions about public health institutions because these cultural values influence the efficiency of these institutions in delivering the optimal benefits for all sections of their societies. Our results about significant association of the four national cultural values with the four socio-economic indicators support the above results, except for a few non-significant findings about some hypothesized relationships.

In fact, our results also address some of the mixed findings reported in the past. For example, Tang and Koveos (2008) find significant relationships between national wealth (per capita GDP) and three of the five national culture dimensions (PDI, IDV, and LTO) but not for UAI and masculinity. Tang and Koveos (2008) explain these results by arguing that UAI and masculinity are relatively stable cultural values in comparison to the other three Hofstede dimensions and hence, these may not be able to explain any changes in national wealth. Our results extend these prior findings by showing a consistent pattern in the impact of the four national cultural dimensions on the four socio-economic indicators. Of course, it would be interesting to see the changes in these results during and after a global health crisis like the ongoing COVID-19, wherein the level of economic output has been affected by frequent lockdowns, travel restrictions, and other factors that may affect national wealth in the short term.

Next, the significant impact of all the four socio-economic indicators on the three public health infrastructure measures confirms the importance of economic development and human welfare (Borisova et al., 2017). Similarly, the significant impact of public health infrastructure on COVID-19 outcomes shows the importance of investing in public health infrastructure to deal with any global health crisis despite the delayed response and mismanagement of public health systems due to unclear policies and priorities in many countries during this crisis, irrespective of their level of socio-economic development (Patterson, 2020; Qato, 2020).

5.12 Conclusion

Despite its potential theoretical contribution and practical implications, this chapter has a few limitations that future research may address. First, our empirical analysis is constrained by the availability of data on Hofstede's national cultural values for only 69 countries; hence, future studies may use other measures or proxies of national culture to fully utilize the data on the other variables in our model that is available for about 200 countries and above. Second, we include only GDPC, HDI, and HEX as indicators for socio-economic development and BEDS, PHYS and TESTS for public health infrastructure. Future research may include other indicators to provide a more comprehensive view of how these variables may be influenced by national cultural values and impact public health outcomes in return. COVID-19 revealed the intricate tapestry of global responses, driven by a complex amalgamation of political, socio-economic, and cultural factors. The pandemic emphasizes that while diverse strategies emerge, the commonality lies in the shared objective of safeguarding public health. As nations reflect on their approaches, the lessons learned and challenges faced pave the way for future cooperation, preparedness, and global health security.

5.13   Future lessons for managers

Overall, this chapter makes some useful theoretical contributions. First, our integrative multi-stage conceptual model combines Hofstede's national cultural framework with the institutional perspective to assess the process by which national cultural values may influence public health outcomes through socio-economic resources and public health infrastructure. With this integrative multi-stage model, we extend the growing research on the role of public institutions and policies in managing public health outcomes, which have been challenged to an extreme by the ongoing COVID-19 (e.g., Hwang & Höllerer, 2020). This study highlights the extent to which governments need to look beyond their existing rigid policies and legal frameworks in order to develop and implement new alternatives to ensure quick deployment and optimal results (Kurdin, 2020). Therefore, we expect this model to guide future research on the management of similar global crises by tapping into the impact of culture on the public institutions that are expected to anticipate and manage the process.

From a practical point of view, this study highlights that it is not sufficient to have a high-income economy that boasts of high level of human development as indicated by popular indicators, nor is it enough to spend a lot of money on creating a massive public health infrastructure (e.g., hospitals, beds, doctors, tests) if it cannot help them recover if they are infected by a new virus or prevent them from dying once they are hospitalized. In fact, COVID-19 has influenced people in so many dramatic ways that it is difficult to imagine the world ever going back to the way it used to be before this crisis, which has included accelerating changes that were already happening albeit at a much slower rate, such as contactless payment systems, online shopping, online education, and telemedicine. More importantly, this pandemic has revealed cracks in our existing institutional arrangements that have been exacerbated by their inherent 'contradictions, heterogeneity, and multiplicity', triggering a move towards transformative changes (Hwang & Höllerer, 2020).

6 COVID-19 business response

Adaptation, resilience, and innovation

6.1 Immediate response of businesses to COVID-19

The immediate response of businesses to COVID-19 showcased resilience, adaptability, and a commitment to safeguarding both employees and the continuity of operations amid unprecedented challenges (Sharma et al., 2020). The strategies employed during this phase often set the foundation for ongoing resilience and recovery efforts, as discussed in this section.

Emergency response planning: Businesses initiated emergency response plans to address the immediate impact of the pandemic. This involved establishing crisis management teams, defining roles and responsibilities, and implementing communication protocols (Liu et al., 2020). *Agility and flexibility:* The ability to quickly adapt and pivot became a crucial aspect of business survival. Companies that demonstrated agility in adjusting their operations, products, or services were better positioned to weather the uncertainties. *Scenario planning:* Scenario planning became essential for businesses to assess the potential impact of different scenarios and plan for various contingencies. This helped businesses anticipate challenges and make informed decisions. *Risk management and compliance:* Businesses focused on risk management, including compliance with evolving health and safety regulations. This involved staying informed about government guidelines, implementing necessary changes, and conducting regular risk assessments (Wang et al., 2023).

Remote work and digital transformation: Many businesses quickly adopted remote work arrangements to comply with lockdowns and social distancing measures. This required a rapid shift to digital technologies, collaboration tools, and cloud-based platforms to enable employees to work from home (Daneshfar et al., 2023). *Employee safety measures:* Businesses implemented safety measures for employees who couldn't work remotely, including enhanced sanitation protocols, social distancing in workplaces, and the provision of personal protective equipment (PPE) where necessary (Daniels et al., 2022). *Communication and employee support:* Clear and transparent communication became essential with employees in order to provide updates on the situation, changes in operations, and support available to them during the pandemic, including mental health resources, employee assistance programs

DOI: 10.4324/9781003227113-7

(EAPs), and flexible work arrangements to support the well-being of their workforce (LaBerge et al., 2020).

Supply chain adjustments: Disruptions to global supply chains prompted businesses to reassess and adapt their supply chain strategies. Some diversified suppliers, built redundancies and focused on local sourcing to mitigate risks. Businesses communicated with suppliers and partners to understand potential disruptions, address challenges, and collaborate on finding solutions. Effective communication with the supply chain was crucial for maintaining continuity (Moosavi et al., 2022). *Financial planning and cost reduction:* Many businesses conducted immediate assessments of their financial positions and cash flow. Cost-cutting measures, including layoffs, furloughs, and salary reductions, were implemented to preserve financial stability (Ashraf, 2020; Sharif et al., 2020). *E-commerce and online presence:* Businesses, especially those in retail and services, accelerated their move to e-commerce and strengthened their online presence by developing or enhancing their online sales channels and digital marketing strategies (Agarwal et al., 2022).

Community engagement: Businesses engaged with their local communities by supporting relief efforts, donating resources, or participating in initiatives to address the broader societal challenges posed by the pandemic (Yi et al., 2023). *Customer communication and experience:* Businesses focused on maintaining and enhancing customer relationships by communicating changes in operations, addressing concerns, and ensuring a positive customer experience, even in challenging circumstances (Farmaki et al., 2022). *Health and safety compliance:* Compliance with health and safety regulations and guidelines became a priority, especially for businesses in essential services as they had to implement measures to ensure the health and safety of their employees and customers (Simpeh & Amoah, 2022). *Government support programs:* Businesses explored and accessed government support programs, grants, and financial aid to mitigate the economic impact of the pandemic. This included initiatives to support employee retention, business continuity, and access to capital (Stiglitz, 2021).

6.2 Supply chain resilience

The pandemic exposed vulnerabilities in global supply chains, prompting companies to reassess and diversify their sourcing strategies, with many businesses trying to enhance supply chain resilience by reducing dependencies on single suppliers and exploring localized sourcing options (Ozdemir et al., 2022). Technological solutions, such as blockchain, were employed to improve transparency and traceability. However, building supply chain resilience is an ongoing process, and the lessons learned during the COVID-19 pandemic have prompted businesses to adopt more proactive and adaptive approaches to supply chain management (Panwar et al., 2022). The emphasis on resilience is likely to remain a key consideration in future supply chain strategies. In this section, we describe key strategies and measures that businesses implemented to build and strengthen supply chain resilience during the COVID-19 pandemic.

Supplier relationship management: Strengthening relationships with suppliers became a priority. Businesses collaborated closely with key suppliers, sharing information, and working together to address challenges. This cooperative approach helped build mutual trust and resilience (Kazancoglu et al., 2022). *Collaboration and information sharing:* Collaborative efforts within industries and supply chain networks were encouraged. Businesses shared information about potential challenges, best practices, and solutions to collectively enhance the resilience of the broader supply chain ecosystem (Kazancoglu et al., 2022). *Risk assessment and scenario planning:* Companies conducted thorough risk assessments to identify potential vulnerabilities in the supply chain. Scenario planning allowed businesses to anticipate various disruptions and develop contingency plans for different scenarios (Moosavi et al., 2022). *Continuous monitoring and learning:* Many businesses implemented continuous monitoring mechanisms to stay informed about the evolving situation. Learning from experiences during the pandemic would help businesses plan and implement ongoing improvements in their supply chain resilience strategies (Panwar et al., 2022).

Flexible and agile supply chains: Supply chains were made more flexible and agile to respond quickly to changing conditions. Businesses implemented measures such as dynamic routing, agile manufacturing processes, and quick adaptation to changes in demand (Moosavi et al., 2022). *Diversification of suppliers:* Businesses sought to diversify their supplier base to reduce dependence on a single source. This involved identifying alternative suppliers and establishing relationships with multiple partners to mitigate the risk of disruptions (Spieske & Birkel, 2021). *Local sourcing and nearshoring:* Some businesses reconsidered global sourcing strategies and explored local or regional suppliers. Nearshoring, or bringing production closer to the point of consumption, was considered to reduce lead times and transportation risks (Panwar et al., 2022). *Inventory management:* To buffer against supply chain disruptions, businesses reevaluated inventory levels. Maintaining strategic stockpiles of critical components or finished goods helped companies better navigate sudden fluctuations in demand or supply chain interruptions (Ozdemir et al., 2022).

Advanced analytics and technology: Businesses leveraged advanced analytics and technology to enhance visibility across the supply chain. This included the use of data analytics, artificial intelligence (AI), and real-time monitoring tools to identify potential disruptions and optimize decision-making (Modgil et al., 2022). *Digitalization and automation:* The adoption of digital technologies and automation improved supply chain efficiency and reduced the reliance on manual processes. This increased the ability to manage disruptions and streamline operations (Modgil et al., 2022). *Redundancy in critical areas:* Building redundancy in critical areas of the supply chain helped ensure continuity. This could involve redundant suppliers, redundant production facilities, or contingency plans for critical logistics routes (Ozdemir et al., 2022). ***Regulatory compliance and contingency planning:*** Staying compliant with regulatory requirements and having robust contingency plans in place became essential. This involved understanding and adhering to changing regulations, particularly those related to health and safety (Uddin et al., 2023).

6.3   Innovation and new business models

Faced with the economic destruction and uncertainty about the future brought by COVID-19, many businesses embraced innovation and explored new business models to adapt to the changing landscape, including new products or services, partnerships, and collaborations, coupled with greater digital transformation and identification of new revenue streams (Bukovska et al., 2021). Amidst the crisis, innovation and adaptability shone through with many companies successfully pivoting their operations to produce essential goods and services. For example, distilleries began manufacturing hand sanitizers, fashion companies produced masks, and tech firms redirected their resources towards contact tracing and telehealth solutions (Chesbrough, 2020). These innovations not only addressed immediate needs but also showcased businesses' ability to adapt and contribute to the collective response (Sharma et al., 2022). To summarize, COVID-19 prompted businesses to rethink and innovate their business models to adapt to the challenges and uncertainties of the crisis. This section describes the many ways in which business model innovation occurred during the pandemic.

E-commerce expansion: Many businesses, especially those in retail, hospitality, and services, accelerated their shift to e-commerce. Traditional brick-and-mortar businesses quickly established or enhanced online platforms to reach customers and maintain sales (Alcedo et al., 2022). ***Subscription services and membership models:*** Subscription-based business models gained popularity during the pandemic. Companies introduced subscription services to offer products or services on a recurring basis, providing a predictable revenue stream and fostering customer loyalty (Luthra, 2021). ***Digital transformation in services:*** Service-oriented businesses embraced digital transformation to deliver services remotely. Virtual consultations, online classes, and digital service platforms became prevalent, allowing businesses to continue serving customers in a socially distant manner (Hai et al., 2021). ***Telehealth and remote healthcare services:*** The healthcare industry witnessed a rapid adoption of telehealth services. Virtual doctor consultations, remote monitoring, and digital health platforms became essential components of the healthcare business model (Bhatt et al., 2020). ***Contactless and curbside services:*** Retailers and restaurants adapted by introducing contactless services, such as curbside pickup and contactless delivery. This minimized physical interactions and provided convenience to customers (Wang et al., 2021).

Flexible and remote work policies: Many businesses revised their work policies to accommodate remote work. This shift in the workforce model allowed companies to tap into a broader talent pool, reduce office costs, and provided employees with greater flexibility (Daneshfar et al., 2023). *Innovations in supply chain and logistics:* Supply chain innovations focused on enhancing resilience and responsiveness. Businesses explored technologies like blockchain for transparency, real-time tracking for better visibility, and automation to streamline processes (Kazancoglu et al., 2022). *Local and sustainable business practices:* The emphasis on local sourcing and sustainability became a key element of business model innovation. Businesses re-evaluated their supply chains, sourcing materials locally, and adopting eco-friendly practices to meet evolving consumer preferences (Mattera et al., 2021). *Virtual events and experiences:* With the limitations on in-person gatherings, businesses in the events and entertainment industry innovated by hosting virtual events and experiences. This included virtual conferences, concerts, and online experiences to engage audiences (Estanyol, 2022). *Remote learning and EdTech:* Educational institutions and businesses in the education sector embraced remote learning resulting in the rise of educational technology (EdTech) platforms and online learning models as a significant innovation (Al-Hunaiyyan et al., 2021).

Health and wellness focus: The focus on health and wellness led to innovations in the fitness industry. Virtual fitness classes, wellness apps, and personalized health services gained popularity as consumers sought ways to stay healthy at home (Wetherall et al., 2022). *Hybrid business models:* Some businesses adopted hybrid models that combine traditional and digital elements. This could involve a mix of in-person and online services, creating a flexible and adaptable approach to business operations (Ramsay, 2020). *Collaborative ecosystems:* Businesses explored collaborative ecosystems and partnerships to enhance their offerings. Collaborations with other businesses, startups, or industry players allowed for shared resources, expertise, and market reach (Bernardo et al., 2021). Overall, business model innovation during the COVID-19 pandemic was driven by the need for adaptability, resilience, and responsiveness to face and cope with the changing market conditions. Businesses that embraced these innovations were often better positioned to navigate the challenges posed by the crisis and position themselves for future growth (Sharma et al., 2022).

6.4 Digital transformation and e-commerce

The pandemic accelerated the digital transformation of industries. Businesses rapidly adopted technology to facilitate remote work, online sales, and customer engagement. E-commerce experienced explosive growth as consumers shifted to online shopping. Companies invested in enhancing their digital presence and infrastructure to adapt to changing consumer behavior. The COVID-19 pandemic accelerated digital transformation initiatives and significantly impacted the landscape of e-commerce. In this section, we describe key trends and developments related to digital transformation and e-commerce during the pandemic.

Remote work adoption: Businesses rapidly adopted remote work technologies and collaboration tools to facilitate remote work for employees. Video conferencing, project management tools, and virtual communication platforms became essential for maintaining business operations (Daneshfar et al., 2023). *Cloud services expansion:* The demand for cloud services surged as businesses sought scalable and flexible solutions for remote work, data storage, and application deployment. Cloud computing became central to supporting digital transformation efforts (Sharma et al., 2023). *Automation and AI integration:* Automation and AI were increasingly integrated into business processes. Automation helped streamline workflows, reduce manual intervention, and enhance efficiency in various sectors (Chernoff & Warman, 2023). *E-commerce optimization:* E-commerce platforms underwent optimization to meet increased demand. Businesses invested in user-friendly interfaces, enhanced security measures, and improved logistics to provide a seamless online shopping experience (Alcedo et al., 2022; Mukherjee, 2020).

Digital customer engagement: Companies intensified their efforts to engage customers through digital channels. Virtual events, webinars, and online customer support became crucial for maintaining connections with clients and consumers (Karpen & Conduit, 2020). *Data analytics for decision-making:* Data analytics played a vital role in decision-making. Businesses leveraged data analytics tools to gain insights into customer behavior, market trends, and operational efficiency, helping inform strategic decisions (Jia et al., 2020). *Cybersecurity measures:* The rise in remote work and increased digital activities prompted a heightened focus on cybersecurity. Businesses invested in robust cybersecurity measures to protect sensitive data and secure remote work environments (Lallie et al., 2021). *Digital health solutions:* The healthcare sector experienced a surge in the adoption of digital health solutions. Telehealth services, remote patient monitoring, and digital health platforms saw increased usage to ensure continuity of care (Alwashmi, 2020). *Supply chain visibility:* Digital technologies were employed to enhance supply chain visibility. Real-time tracking, IoT devices, and data analytics helped businesses monitor and optimize their supply chain processes (Moosavi et al., 2022; Ozdemir et al., 2022; Panwar et al., 2022).

Acceleration of online shopping: The pandemic accelerated the shift to online shopping as consumers sought to minimize in-person interactions. E-commerce platforms experienced a significant increase in traffic and transactions (Alcedo et al., 2022; Mukherjee, 2020). *Contactless payments:* Contactless payment methods gained prominence as consumers prioritized safety. Mobile payments, digital wallets, and contactless card transactions became more widely accepted and adopted (World Bank, 2022). *Expansion of delivery services:* Businesses expanded their delivery services to meet increased demand. Same-day delivery, curbside pickup, and other contactless delivery options gained popularity as consumers sought convenience and safety (Wang et al., 2021). *Social commerce growth:* Social media platforms increasingly became e-commerce hubs. Social commerce, where users can purchase products directly within social media apps, saw significant growth (Sheikh et al., 2023).

Personalization and AI usage: E-commerce platforms utilized AI for personalized shopping experiences, with AI-driven recommendations, chatbots for customer support, and virtual try-on features being used to enhance online customer experience (Agarwal et al., 2022). *Subscription services:* Subscription-based models gained traction. Subscription boxes, streaming services, and other subscription-based offerings provided a recurring revenue stream for businesses (Luthra, 2021). *Local and sustainable e-commerce:* There was a growing interest in supporting local businesses and sustainable practices. Consumers sought out local and eco-friendly products through online platforms (Alcedo et al., 2022; Mukherjee, 2020). *Digital marketing strategies:* Businesses adapted their marketing strategies to the rapidly evolving digital landscape by using influencer marketing, social media advertising, and targeted online campaigns to reach their consumers (Jaafar & Khan, 2022). All these changes highlight the importance of digital transformation in helping businesses position themselves to adapt to the new normal and meet the changing expectations of consumers.

6.5   Employee well-being

COVID-19 brought about unprecedented challenges that significantly impacted employee well-being. Businesses and organizations took various measures to support and prioritize the health and well-being of their employees during these challenging times as it became a central concern for them during the COVID-19 pandemic (Wong et al., 2021). Most businesses recognized the importance of employee well-being as they implemented remote work and flexible scheduling. To address this, they introduced mental health support, COVID-19 testing, and vaccination initiatives to ensure the safety and mental health of employees (Hamouche, 2020). Companies that prioritized employee welfare gained not only loyalty but also increased productivity. Strategies to support employees encompassed physical health, mental health, and overall work-life balance, with a recognition of the unique challenges posed by the unprecedented circumstances (Wong et al., 2021). In this section, we describe some key aspects of employee well-being during the pandemic, including its antecedents and outcomes.

Remote work and flexible schedules: Many organizations transitioned to remote work to ensure employee safety. Providing the necessary tools and infrastructure for remote work became a priority. Businesses introduced flexible work hours to accommodate employees dealing with caregiving responsibilities, homeschooling, or other challenges (Daneshfar et al., 2023). *Mental health support:* Companies increased access to mental health resources, including EAPs, counseling services, and online mental health platforms (Wang

et al., 2022b). *Awareness campaigns:* Employers conducted awareness campaigns to reduce the stigma associated with mental health issues and encourage open conversations about well-being (Gualano et al., 2022). *Health and
safety measures:* Employers implemented strict health protocols in physical
workplaces, including temperature checks, sanitation measures, and social
distancing – to ensure the safety of on-site employees. Many businesses provided PPE and hygiene supplies to employees working on-site (Simpeh &
Amoah, 2022). *Communication and transparency:* Maintaining transparent
and regular communication became crucial and most employers kept their
employees informed about the evolving situation, company policies, and
plans for returning to the workplace, using virtual town hall meetings or
communication forums to address employee concerns and questions (Yue &
Walden, 2023).

Financial support: Most employers sought to maintain salary and benefits
continuity, even if adjustments were necessary, and provided clear communication about any changes in compensation or benefits. Some organizations
also introduced their own financial assistance programs or relief funds to
support employees facing economic challenges (Daniels et al., 2022). *EAPs:*
The utilization and expansion of EAPs, offering counseling services, mental
health support, and resources for personal challenges, became more widespread (Daniels et al., 2022). *Training and skill development:* Many employers provided upskilling and professional development to keep their employees
engaged and motivated during periods of remote work. Training programs
were also adapted to virtual formats to accommodate remote work scenarios
(Chun et al., 2021).

Flexible leave and work policies: Flexible leave policies were implemented
to accommodate employees who needed time off due to illness, caregiving
responsibilities, or other pandemic-related challenges. Most businesses also
allowed high-risk individuals to continue working remotely to ensure their
safety (Daneshfar et al., 2023). *Social connection and team building:* Many
employers organized virtual team-building activities to foster social connections among remote teams. Virtual social events, such as virtual happy hours,
game nights, and coffee breaks, were organized to maintain a sense of community (Graham et al., 2023). *Recognition and appreciation:* Recognizing
and appreciating employees' efforts and dedication became a focus. Virtual
recognition events, shout-outs, and appreciation emails were commonly used.
Many companies organized virtual employee appreciation events to celebrate
achievements and boost morale (Qin & Men, 2023).

Employee surveys and feedback: Regular employee surveys and feedback
mechanisms were implemented to understand the specific needs and concerns
of employees. Employers used the feedback to make actionable responses,
addressing concerns and improving workplace policies (Qin & Men, 2023).
Flexibility and compassion: Many employers demonstrated flexibility and
compassion, as their employees navigated personal challenges. Acknowledging the unique circumstances of each employee became a priority (Daneshfar

et al., 2023). ***Return-to-work transition support:*** As some employees returned to the workplace, companies implemented phased return strategies and clear guidelines to ensure a smooth transition. Special attention was given to providing mental health support during transitions back to the workplace (Wang et al., 2022b). ***Employee well-being initiatives:*** Many employers initiated well-being programs focusing on employee well-being, including fitness challenges, mindfulness sessions, and well-being workshops (Andrulli & Gerards, 2023).

6.6 Community engagement and corporate social responsibility (CSR)

During the COVID-19 pandemic, community engagement and CSR took on increased significance as businesses sought to support their communities and address the broader societal impact of the crisis (Beninger & Francis, 2022). For example, many businesses engaged with their communities during the pandemic through donations of funds, PPE, and meals to healthcare workers and vulnerable populations, to demonstrate their CSR, which in turn helped them strengthen their relationships with communities and bolstered their brand reputation (Farmaki et al., 2022). In this section, we describe several ways in which companies engaged with their communities and demonstrated CSR during the pandemic.

Donations and philanthropy: Many companies donated funds to support COVID-19 relief efforts. These funds were directed toward healthcare infrastructure, medical supplies, and support for vulnerable populations. Some businesses also contributed essential products, such as PPE, hand sanitizers, and hygiene supplies, to healthcare facilities and frontline workers (Zhang & Wang, 2022). ***Employee volunteerism***: Many employers encouraged and supported their employees to volunteer by giving them opportunities to contribute their time and skills to community organizations or participate in virtual volunteering initiatives (Aguinis et al., 2020; Lachance, 2021).

Support for healthcare workers: Businesses offered support services to healthcare workers, such as free meals, transportation assistance, and accommodations to reduce the burden on those working tirelessly on the front lines. Recognizing the mental health challenges faced by healthcare workers, some companies provided mental health resources, counseling services, and well-being programs (Vizheh et al., 2020). ***Small business support:*** Many large companies provided financial assistance and support programs to local small businesses that were particularly affected by lockdowns and restrictions (Katare et al., 2021). Collaborations with local businesses and initiatives aimed at boosting entrepreneurship were also launched by many large corporates to support economic recovery at the community level and contribute to CSR efforts (Islam et al., 2023).

Education and digital inclusion: Some businesses focused on supporting education, particularly remote learning initiatives, including donations of devices, internet connectivity solutions, and educational resources for students (Dorn et al., 2021). Many companies also engaged in digital literacy programs to bridge the digital divide and ensure that communities had the skills needed for remote work and education (Wardana et al., 2023). *Food security initiatives:* Many businesses contributed to food banks and community pantries to address food insecurity exacerbated by the economic impact of the pandemic. Some companies initiated meal programs, providing free or discounted meals to individuals and families facing financial difficulties (Mahmud et al., 2021).

Communication and awareness campaigns: Companies engaged in public health messaging, leveraging their communication channels to disseminate accurate information about COVID-19 prevention and safety measures. Community awareness campaigns focused on issues such as mental health, domestic violence, and community resilience were launched to provide valuable information and resources (Kharbat et al., 2023). *Sustainable practices and environmental initiatives:* Companies continued to prioritize sustainability and environmental responsibility. Some launched initiatives to reduce environmental impact and promote sustainable practices (Mattera et al., 2021). For example, many businesses engaged in green initiatives, such as tree planting, to contribute to environmental conservation efforts.

Support for vulnerable populations: Efforts were made to support vulnerable populations, including the elderly, refugees, and people experiencing homelessness (Patel et al., 2020a). Companies provided assistance through financial support, essential supplies, and shelter programs (Raimo et al., 2021). Collaborations with non-governmental organizations (NGOs) and community-based organizations were established to address the specific needs of marginalized communities. *Continued employment and employee well-being:* Many employers prioritized the well-being of their own employees with measures such as mental health support, flexible work arrangements, and EAPs being implemented (Andrulli & Gerards, 2023). Maintaining job security and minimizing layoffs were key aspects of CSR during a time of economic uncertainty.

Collaboration with governments and health authorities: Businesses collaborated with local governments, health authorities, and international organizations to align their efforts with broader public health and safety initiatives. Ensuring compliance with public health regulations and guidelines became a crucial aspect of CSR (Bernardo et al., 2021; Liu et al., 2020). *Transparent reporting and accountability:* Companies engaged in transparent reporting of their CSR initiatives, detailing their contributions to communities and the impact of their efforts. Establishing accountability measures and reporting mechanisms demonstrated commitment to transparency and responsible business practices (Yue & Walden, 2023). CSR during the pandemic extended beyond immediate business concerns to address the well-being of communities and society at large (Zhang & Wang, 2022). The initiatives undertaken by businesses aimed to provide meaningful support and contribute to the collective resilience and recovery efforts (Chang et al., 2022; Stiglitz, 2021; Wang et al., 2023).

6.7 Financial resilience for individuals, businesses, and governments

Financial resilience became a critical focus for individuals, businesses, and governments as they navigated the economic challenges triggered by the pandemic (Danisman et al., 2021). Companies revised financial models, cut non-essential expenses, and sought government aid to weather the economic downturn, while others diversified revenue streams to reduce reliance on a single source of income (Cheema-Fox et al., 2021). Similarly, individuals cut down discretionary expenditures and increased their savings (Lusardi et al. 2021), while governments provided an economic stimulus to keep their economies alive and financial support to help individuals and households cope with the pandemic (Ashraf, 2020; Delardas et al., 2022). In this section, we describe the key strategies and measures employed by individuals, businesses, and governments, to enhance financial resilience during the pandemic.

Individuals: Individuals prioritized building and maintaining emergency savings to cover essential expenses in case of job loss or unexpected financial setbacks (Sun et al., 2022). For example, people revisited their household budgets to cut non-essential expenses and redirect funds to essential items. Monitoring and adjusting spending patterns became crucial for financial stability (Belletsky et al., 2020). Individuals reached out to creditors and lenders to negotiate payment terms or explore debt relief options and seek refinancing opportunities to reduce monthly debt obligations (Mehdipanah, 2020). People also sought advice from financial advisors and financial planners to assess their situation, set realistic goals, and plan for the future (Fox & Bartholomae, 2020). Some individuals used the time during lockdowns to upskill or reskill, enhancing their professional capabilities and making themselves more marketable in a challenging job market (Falkner et al., 2022). Exploring new career paths and opportunities, and considering diversification in skill sets, became part of a proactive approach to financial resilience. Individuals reviewed their health insurance coverage and considered additional protection measures to safeguard against potential medical expenses. People also explored and utilized government assistance programs, unemployment benefits, and other financial relief measures to mitigate the economic impact of the pandemic (Mansour, 2022).

Businesses: Businesses focused on maintaining healthy cash reserves to withstand economic uncertainties as cash flow management became a priority for their short-term stability (Chang et al., 2020). Companies also implemented cost reduction strategies, including layoffs, furloughs, salary cuts, and other measures to preserve financial stability (Chang et al., 2020). Businesses also explored diversification of products, services, or customer segments to reduce reliance on a single revenue source, and thus, innovating products, services, or business models allowed some companies to adapt to changing market dynamics and meet new demands (Ino & Watanabe, 2022). Companies reassessed and strengthened their supply chains, considering diversification of suppliers, building redundancy, and leveraging technology for better visibility (Kazancoglu et al., 2022). Businesses could transition to remote work arrangements, reducing overhead costs associated with physical offices and ensuring continuity of operations (Daneshfar et al., 2023). Businesses also explored and accessed a diverse range of government support programs wherever available, including grants, loans, and stimulus packages – to ease financial pressures and sustain operations (Cirera et al., 2021).

Businesses focused on maintaining strong relationships with existing customers using regular communication, customer support, and loyalty programs to retain customer trust (Kumar, 2022). The pandemic also accelerated digital transformation initiatives with many businesses investing in emerging technologies to enhance their online presence, e-commerce capabilities, and digital customer engagement (Hai et al., 2021). Companies engaged in scenario planning to anticipate potential challenges and formulate strategies for different economic scenarios and implemented robust risk management practices to identify and mitigate potential risks to their business (Wang et al., 2023). Companies recognized the importance of supporting employee well-being with initiatives such as mental health programs, flexible work arrangements, and EAPs (Wong et al., 2021).

Governments: Most governments introduced economic stimulus packages to support businesses and individuals and provide financial relief to boost economic activity and unemployment benefits to help individuals who lost their jobs during the pandemic (Augustin et al., 2022). Governments also allocated funds to strengthen healthcare systems, invest in medical infrastructure, and procure essential medical supplies. Many governments also offered tax relief measures, such as deferrals, credits, and reductions – to ease the financial burden on businesses and individuals (Sharif et al., 2020). Some governments implemented debt moratoriums, allowing individuals and businesses to defer loan repayments during challenging periods (Stiglitz, 2021). Governments expanded social welfare programs to provide support to vulnerable populations facing financial hardships and invested in digital inclusion initiatives to bridge the digital divide and ensure that all segments of the population could access essential services online (Mittal et al., 2022). Governments also adopted regulatory flexibility measures to accommodate the diverse circumstances and challenges facing different segments of their populations (Taylor et al., 2020).

6.8   Hybrid work models

The pandemic reshaped the future of work, with the rise of hybrid work models, which combine remote work and in-person work (Verma et al., 2023). Companies recognized that remote work was viable and offered flexibility, which became an attractive option for employees reeling under the devastating impact of the pandemic (Daneshfar et al., 2023). Businesses began re-evaluating their office spaces and work policies to accommodate these changes as hybrid work models became increasingly popular during the COVID-19 pandemic as organizations adapted to the challenges posed by the crisis (Verma et al., 2023). In this section, we describe the key aspects and considerations of hybrid work models implemented during the pandemic.

Remote work and flexible arrangements: Hybrid work models allowed employees to work remotely for part of the week while spending the remaining time working in the office. Employees often had the flexibility to choose their workdays in the office and remote workdays based on their preferences and job requirements (Daneshfar et al., 2023). *Digital collaboration and transformation:* Most organizations invested in and relied heavily on digital collaboration tools, such as video conferencing, project management platforms, and communication apps, to facilitate seamless collaboration among remote and in-office teams (Wardana et al., 2023). Cloud-based systems and technologies were implemented to ensure that employees could access necessary resources and information from any location (Sharma et al., 2023). *Workspace redesign and adaptation:* Offices were redesigned to accommodate flexible work arrangements, which included creating open collaboration spaces, hot desking options, and technology-enabled meeting rooms (Chang et al., 2022).

Health and safety measures: Organizations implemented health and safety measures in the office, such as social distancing protocols, and increased sanitation practices and touchless technology to minimize physical contact (Simpeh & Amoah, 2022). *Employee well-being and work-life balance:* Hybrid work models aimed to support better work-life balance by reducing commuting time and providing more flexibility in managing personal and professional commitments (Wong et al., 2021). *Mental health support:* Employers recognized the importance of supporting employee mental health in hybrid work environments, offering resources, counseling services, and initiatives to combat remote work-related challenges (Andrulli & Gerards, 2023). *Clear communication and transparent policies:* Organizations established clear and transparent policies and guidelines on work hours, communication norms, and in-office attendance requirements (Kharbat et al., 2023). Regular communication from leadership and HR teams provided updates on the evolving situation, changes in policies, and the organization's commitment to employee well-being (Qin & Men, 2023).

Collaboration and team building: Organizations encouraged both virtual and in-person collaboration by organizing team-building activities and virtual social events to foster a sense of community among remote and in-office employees (Wardana et al., 2023). Meetings were designed to accommodate both remote and in-person participants, leveraging technology to ensure equal participation and engagement (Jaafar & Khan, 2022). *Performance measurement:* Rather than focusing solely on hours worked, organizations shifted toward outcome-based performance evaluation. This approach emphasized productivity, results, and contributions to team goals (Narayanamurthy &

Tortorella, 2021). ***Regular check-ins:*** Regular check-ins between managers and employees helped track progress, address challenges, and ensure that employees felt supported in their roles (Kaushik & Guleria, 2020).

Training and upskilling: Organizations invested in training programs to enhance digital skills for both remote and in-office work, by upskilling employees in the use of collaboration tools and remote work technologies (Falkner et al., 2022). ***Continuous learning:*** Continuous learning initiatives were promoted to ensure that employees stayed updated on industry trends and developments (Adedoyin & Soykan, 2023). ***Inclusive leadership:*** Organizations emphasized inclusive leadership to ensure that all employees, regardless of their work location, received equitable treatment, opportunities for career growth, and access to resources (Ahmed et al., 2020). ***Mitigating inequities:*** Efforts were made to mitigate potential inequities between remote and in-office workers, ensuring that everyone felt connected and valued (Fortier, 2020).

Flexibility and Adaptability: Hybrid work models required organizations and employees to be adaptable to change by adjusting to evolving circumstances, using feedback mechanisms for continuous improvement, and staying agile in response to emerging needs (Wong et al., 2021). ***Policy development and compliance:*** Organizations developed flexible policies that allowed for adjustments based on the evolving situation, including considerations for changes in public health guidelines, government regulations, and employee preferences (Liu et al., 2020). ***Legal and compliance considerations:*** Compliance with labor laws, data protection regulations, and other legal considerations were addressed in the development of hybrid work policies (Bernardo et al., 2021). Although hybrid work models evolved as a response to the dynamic challenges posed by the COVID-19 pandemic, the success of these models often depended on effective communication, technology enablement, and a commitment to employee well-being and inclusivity (Verma et al., 2023).

6.9   Conclusion

The business response to COVID-19 exemplified adaptability, resilience, and innovation in the face of extraordinary challenges. The pandemic accelerated digital transformation, reshaped supply chain strategies, and prioritized employee well-being. It emphasized the importance of CSR and financial resilience. As businesses move forward, the lessons learned during this crisis will continue to inform strategies for navigating an unpredictable and evolving global landscape. As shown in Figure 6.1, organizations that showed resilience during COVID-19 displayed a few common characteristics. First, they were able to quickly establish a common purpose and clear communications to deal with the pandemic and its impact on their customers, employees, and other stakeholders. Second, they were able to set up structures that allowed rapid decision-making without any bureaucratic delays. Third, they could create and leverage the knowledge and reach of their networks of local teams with clear and accountable roles. Fourth, they developed a culture that trusted

1	2	3	4	5
Establish a common purpose and clear communications	Set up structures to allow rapid decision making	Create networks of local teams with clear, accountable roles	Develop a culture that empowers people	Provide people with the technology they need
• Develop a common purpose that holds true in peacetime and focus on more frequent communications with employees	• Retain the rapid-decision-making cycles implemented during the COVID-19 crisis, but in a way that ensures long-term sustainability	• Continue to develop networks of local teams and business units, encouraging sharing of lessons learned and best practices between them	• Ensure people continue to feel empowered, rather than returning to central control and rigid processes, and invest in leadership that develops people	• Consider which new technologies to embed in ongoing ways of working
• Agile organizations often speak of a shared purpose and vision—the "North Star"—which helps people feel personally invested in the company	• Agile organizations emphasize quick, efficient, and continuous decision making, rather than making big bets	• Agile organizations go beyond empowering local teams to creating dense networks of teams with clear, flat structures	• In agile organizations, leaders act as visionaries, architects, and coaches	• Agile organizations seamlessly integrate technology—it is core to every aspect of the organization

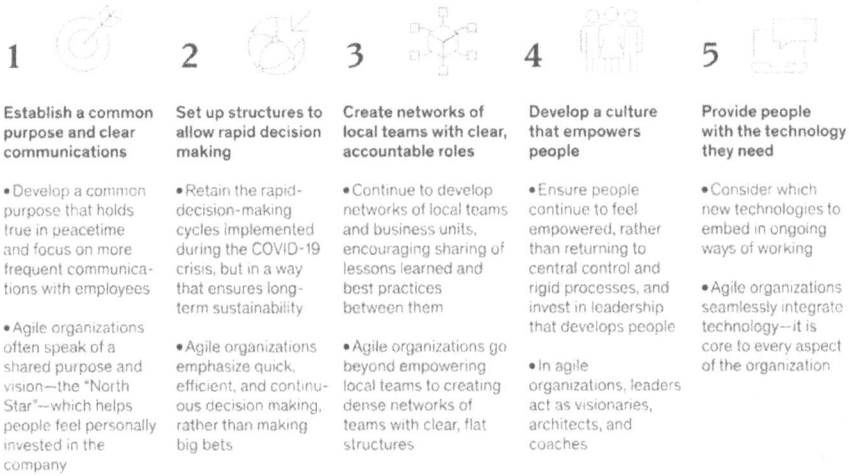

Figure 6.1 Common characteristics displayed by resilient organizations during COVID-19

Source: McKinsey & Company (https://www.mckinsey.com/capabilities/people-and-organizational-performance/our-insights)

and empowered their employees. Finally, they were able to quickly adopt new technologies to enable their employees to continue serving their customers in the most effective manner.

6.10   Future lessons for managers

As organizations continue to navigate the aftermath of the COVID-19 pandemic, there are several key lessons for managers to enhance adaptation, resilience, and innovation. These lessons are designed to help organizations not only recover from the impacts of the pandemic but also thrive in an ever-changing and uncertain environment. First and foremost, managers need to foster agile leadership styles that emphasize adaptability, quick decision-making, and the ability to navigate ambiguity. Leaders should be comfortable with experimentation and learning from failures as demonstrated by their collective experiences during the pandemic. This process would be helped to a great extent by cultivating a culture of continuous learning within the organization, such as encouraging employees to acquire new skills and stay updated on industry trends, which in turn would enhance the organization's ability to adapt to rapidly changing and evolving circumstances. Organizations should also continue to invest in emerging technologies to improve their efficiency through collaboration and innovation, which would require no hesitation in embracing digital transformation, in order to stay competitive and resilient in a rapidly changing business landscape and tackle unexpected shocks.

Managers should also build on the learnings from the experiences with remote work during the pandemic by developing and refining flexible work models, which may involve hybrid work arrangements that allow employees to work both remotely in a virtual mode and in a physical office in an in-person mode. Similarly, managers should recognize the value of diverse perspectives and inclusive decision-making by encouraging diversity, equity, and inclusion in their teams to make them more innovative and better equipped to tackle complex challenges (Jones et al., 2023). All these efforts should be further supported by ensuring employee well-being which is necessary to foster a healthy and engaged workforce, by providing mental health support, flexible work arrangements, and initiatives to promote work-life balance. All of these are necessary steps towards building a more robust and resilient workforce.

Organizations should also improve their supply chain resilience by diversifying suppliers and creating redundancy in critical supply chain components, which would help them mitigate the risks associated with any unanticipated and undesirable disruptions in their supply chains. This can be ensured by developing robust scenario planning and risk management processes to anticipate potential challenges and have contingency plans in place to respond effectively to various scenarios. Managers should also encourage collaboration across different departments and functions within the organization by breaking down silos – to facilitate communication and information-sharing, fostering a more integrated and responsive organizational structure. Managers should also form strategic partnerships with other organizations to share resources, knowledge, and expertise, as such collaborative efforts can help them enhance their resilience and foster a culture of innovation. Organizations should also aim to innovate with a focus on meeting evolving customer needs, by soliciting customer feedback, leveraging customer data, and developing new products and services based on customer preferences and expectations.

Managers should also embrace sustainability and social responsibility as integral parts of their strategies, as focusing on environmental and social issues can provide a better connection with the broader society and contribute to long-term resilience and innovation. To achieve these goals, managers should stay informed about the latest economic and geopolitical developments that may impact their organizations, as it would help them make strategic decisions by anticipating potential challenges and opportunities. Managers should also continue to prioritize clear and transparent communication with their employees, customers, suppliers, investors, and other key stakeholders, to build trust and manage expectations during times of change or crisis. Finally, managers should develop governance structures that are adaptive to change, help them make decisions quickly, reassess strategies regularly, and adjust organizational priorities as needed. All these lessons can serve as a foundation for managers seeking to enhance their organizations' ability to adapt, remain resilient, and foster innovation in the post-COVID-19 era.

7 COVID-19 important management lessons
Learning from failures

7.1 Agility and adaptability

COVID-19 highlighted the importance of agility and adaptability in organizational operations to help businesses navigate unforeseen challenges and uncertainties, wherein rigid business models and processes quickly became obsolete in the face of large-scale and wide-spread disruptions (Elali, 2021). Companies that were able to pivot their strategies, products, and services in response to the changing landscape fared better during the crisis, which underscores the need for managers to foster a culture that encourages innovation, flexibility, and the willingness to embrace change (Hamilton, 2020). As the business landscape continues to evolve in the post-COVID-19 era, these qualities remain crucial for sustained success. In this section, we discuss the key reasons why agility and adaptability are important for businesses.

Rapid response to changing market dynamics: The post-COVID-19 environment is marked by rapid changes in consumer behavior, market demands, and economic conditions. Agile businesses can quickly respond to these changes, adjusting their strategies and operations accordingly (Dahlke et al., 2021). *Navigating economic and global uncertainties:* The pandemic has introduced a level of economic and global uncertainty. Agile businesses are better equipped to navigate uncertainties, make informed decisions, and adjust their plans as needed (Sharma et al., 2020). *Continuous innovation and creativity:* Adaptability fosters a culture of continuous innovation. Businesses that prioritize adaptability are more likely to embrace new ideas, technologies, and business models to stay ahead in the market (Bukovska et al., 2021). *Data-driven decision-making:* Agile businesses leverage data-driven insights to inform decision-making. The ability to analyze and act upon data quickly is a hallmark of adaptability in a rapidly changing business environment (Jia et al., 2020). *Accelerated digital adoption and transformation:* The pandemic accelerated digital transformation across industries (OECD, 2020b). Agile businesses are better positioned to leverage new technologies, embrace digital solutions, and stay ahead in the era of digital business (Hai et al., 2021).

Customer-centric approaches: With the changing consumer preferences and behaviors during and after the pandemic, agile businesses are paying more

DOI: 10.4324/9781003227113-8

attention to these changes and are responding proactively by tailoring their products, services, and customer experiences accordingly (Karpen & Conduit, 2020). *Responsive customer service:* Rapid adaptation ensures that businesses can address customer concerns, feedback, and changing expectations promptly. This responsiveness contributes to customer satisfaction and retention (Rabiul et al., 2022). *Customer trust and brand reputation:* Businesses that adapt and communicate transparently during times of change build and maintain customer trust. A strong brand reputation is often associated with a company's ability to navigate challenges effectively (Farmaki et al., 2022). *Employee engagement and well-being:* Post-COVID-19 era is experiencing a continuation of remote and hybrid work models. Agility is vital for businesses to create flexible work environments that support employee well-being, satisfaction, and productivity (Wong et al., 2021). *Talent attraction and retention:* A culture of adaptability is attractive to top talent. Businesses that foster an adaptable work culture are more likely to attract and retain skilled professionals who value innovation and resilience (Stiglitz, 2021).

Supply chain and operational challenges: The pandemic exposed vulnerabilities in supply chains and operations. Adaptability allows businesses to build resilience, reconfigure supply chains, and implement contingency plans to address operational challenges (Kazancoglu et al., 2022). *Competitive advantage:* Quick adaptation to changing market conditions allows businesses to seize opportunities and enter new markets more effectively. This agility can lead to a competitive advantage over slower-moving competitors (Mahdi & Nassar, 2021). *Proactive risk mitigation:* The ability to adapt quickly is crucial for proactive risk management. Agile businesses can identify, assess, and mitigate risks more effectively, reducing the impact of potential disruptions (Wang et al., 2023). *Regulatory compliance:* In post-COVID-19 period, regulatory landscapes may change. Businesses need to be agile in understanding and complying with evolving regulations, ensuring they remain in good standing with legal requirements (Uddin et al., 2023). *Sustainable business practices:* Adaptability as a business characteristic naturally extends to sustainable business practices. Businesses that can adapt their operations to align with environmental and social considerations are more likely to meet evolving consumer expectations (Mattera et al., 2021).

Overall, in the post-COVID-19 landscape, where change is likely to be the only constant, businesses that prioritize agility and adaptability are better positioned to thrive, innovate, and meet the dynamic needs of their customers and stakeholders (Bullock et al., 2022). The ability to pivot quickly, embrace change, and learn from experiences will be essential for long-term success (Kazancoglu et al., 2022; Panwar et al., 2022; Stiglitz, 2021).

7.2   Remote work and technology

The COVID-19 pandemic has significantly accelerated the adoption of remote work and use of new technologies across industries and even with the pandemic having subsided, the impact on how we work and the use of technology is likely to persist (Narayanamurthy & Tortorella, 2021). Managers have learned that remote work is not only feasible but can also enhance productivity and work-life balance with virtual collaboration tools having become lifelines for businesses, enabling teams to continue working seamlessly (Hai et al., 2021). This experience has underscored the importance of investing in robust technological infrastructure and digital literacy, and managers should recognize that the future of work might involve hybrid models that blend remote and in-office operations (Daneshfar et al., 2023). In this section, we describe key post-COVID-19 trends and considerations related to remote work and technology.

Hybrid work models: Many organizations are adopting hybrid work models, allowing employees to work both remotely and in the office. This flexibility provides a balance between the benefits of remote work and the advantages of in-person collaboration (Verma et al., 2023). ***Remote work as a permanent feature:*** Some companies have embraced remote work as a permanent or long-term feature of their business model to allow them access to a broader talent pool and reduce the need for physical office space (Daneshfar et al., 2023). ***Persistent reliance on collaboration platforms:*** The use of digital collaboration tools, such as video conferencing, project management, and communication platforms, will continue to be a staple in facilitating remote work and enhancing team collaboration (Wardana et al., 2023). ***Technology infrastructure investment:*** Organizations will continue to invest in robust IT infrastructure to support remote work securely. This includes cloud computing, cybersecurity measures, and technologies that enable seamless communication and collaboration (Hai et al., 2021). ***Heightened cybersecurity protocols:*** As remote work introduces new cybersecurity challenges, organizations will invest in advanced cybersecurity measures to protect sensitive data and ensure the security of remote work environments (Lallie et al., 2021).

Focus on employee well-being and mental health support: Companies will increasingly prioritize employee well-being in remote work settings. Initiatives related to mental health support, work-life balance, and virtual team-building activities will be integral to continued business success (Wong et al., 2021). ***Digital skills development:*** To support remote work, there will be a continued emphasis on training and upskilling employees in digital competencies, which includes proficiency in digital collaboration tools, cybersecurity awareness, and other relevant skills (Hai et al., 2021). ***Virtual onboarding and integration:*** Remote work will influence the way new employees are onboarded, using virtual onboarding processes, including video introductions, digital training modules, and virtual mentorship, will become more common (Wong et al., 2021). ***Emergence of virtual collaboration tools:*** Continued innovation in virtual collaboration tools will facilitate more immersive and effective online meetings, brainstorming sessions, and project collaboration (Hai et al., 2021).

Employee monitoring to balance productivity and privacy: The use of employee monitoring tools will continue to be a topic of discussion as employers will need to strike a balance between monitoring productivity and respecting employee privacy (Blumenfeld et al., 2020). ***Formalization of remote work policies:*** Organizations will establish and formalize remote work policies to provide clear guidelines on expectations, communication norms, and performance evaluation for remote and hybrid work arrangements (Daneshfar et al., 2023). ***Virtual and inclusive culture:*** Companies will work to foster an inclusive workplace culture that spans virtual and in-person interactions. Initiatives to maintain a sense of community and shared values will be crucial (Eikhof, 2020). ***Adaptive work schedules:*** Flexible work hours will become more standard. Employees will have the freedom to set work hours that align with their personal preferences, contributing to improved work-life balance (LaBerge et al., 2020; Sangster Jokić & Jokić-Begić, 2022).

Global talent pool access: Remote work would allow businesses to tap into a global talent pool. Companies may continue to recruit talent without geographical restrictions, promoting diversity and expertise within teams (Daneshfar et al., 2023). ***Rise of digital nomad workforce:*** Remote work allows employees to work from anywhere. This has given rise to the concept of digital nomadism, where individuals can choose to work from different locations, including international destinations (Daneshfar et al., 2023). ***Adaptive leadership styles:*** Leadership styles will adapt to manage remote and hybrid teams as leaders will need to focus on communication, empathy, and creating a sense of purpose in a virtual environment in the post-COVID-19 era (Ahmed et al., 2020, Qin & Men, 2023).

Demand for remote work solutions: The technology industry will experience sustained demand for remote work solutions, including tools for virtual collaboration, cybersecurity, and innovations that enhance the remote work experience (Daneshfar et al., 2023). ***Sustainability considerations:*** Remote work contributes to a reduction in commuting and office energy consumption. Companies may consider sustainability initiatives and reduce their environmental impact with a distributed workforce (Mattera et al., 2021). ***Regulatory and legal considerations:*** Companies will navigate evolving regulations related to remote work, including compliance with labor laws, data protection, and remote work taxation (Uddin et al., 2023). ***Customer-centric digital experiences:*** Businesses will continue to enhance digital customer experiences, leveraging technology for online engagement, e-commerce, and customer support (Karpen et al., 2020). Overall, the post-COVID-19 era will see a transformation in how businesses approach work and technology. The lessons learned during the pandemic will shape a more adaptable, technology-driven, and employee-centric future. Organizations that embrace these changes are likely to thrive in the evolving landscape.

7.3   Employee well-being and empathy

The pandemic brought to the forefront the significance of employee well-being and mental health as managers realized that a supportive and empathetic approach towards their teams is vital (Wong et al., 2021). The crisis blurred the lines between work and personal life, leading to burnout and stress. Going forward, managers need to prioritize creating a work environment that promotes work-life balance, offers mental health resources, and fosters open communication (Sangster Jokić & Jokić-Begić, 2022). Employee well-being and empathy have gained increased recognition as crucial elements of a healthy and productive work environment, especially in the post-COVID-19 era (Wong et al., 2021). In this section, we discuss the key considerations for employee well-being and empathy in the post-COVID-19 workplace.

Flexible work arrangements: Offering flexibility in work arrangements, including hybrid and remote work options, supports employee well-being by allowing for a better balance between professional and personal responsibilities (LaBerge et al., 2020). *Access to mental health resources:* Providing access to mental health resources, counseling services, and educational materials helps employees manage stress, anxiety, and other mental health challenges. Fostering a culture that reduces the stigma associated with mental health concerns would also encourage employees to seek help when needed (Sangster Jokić & Jokić-Begić, 2022). *Empathetic leadership:* Leaders who demonstrate empathy understand the unique needs and challenges faced by their employees. This includes recognizing personal situations, providing support, and showing a genuine interest in their well-being (Ahmed et al., 2020). *Open and transparent communication:* Communicating openly about organizational changes, challenges, and successes contributes to a sense of trust and reduces uncertainty (Kharbat et al., 2023). Establishing regular feedback mechanisms would allow employees to voice concerns, provide input, and feel valued in the decision-making process (Qin & Men, 2023).

Work-life balance: Encouraging employees to set clear boundaries between work and personal life would promote a healthier work-life balance, which includes respecting non-working hours and providing the flexibility needed to maintain personal well-being (LaBerge et al., 2020). *Recognition and appreciation:* Recognizing and appreciating employee efforts and achievements contribute to a positive work environment, through verbal recognition, awards, or other forms of acknowledgment (Wong et al., 2021). *Building resilience:* Offering training programs on resilience helps employees develop coping mechanisms to navigate challenges and setbacks, contributing to long-term well-being (Chang et al., 2022). *Inclusive work environment:* Fostering an inclusive work environment where employees feel valued and respected for their unique perspectives and backgrounds contributes to overall well-being (Eikhof, 2020). *Team building and social connections:* Encouraging team-building activities, whether virtual or in-person, helps build social connections and a sense of camaraderie among team members (Graham et al., 2023). *Celebrating milestones:* Celebrating personal and professional milestones fosters a positive and supportive workplace culture (Qin & Men, 2023).

Employee Assistance Programs (EAPs): Implementing or expanding EAPs provides employees with access to counseling services, financial advice, and other support resources (Andrulli & Gerards, 2023). *Health and wellness initiatives:* Implementing wellness programs, fitness challenges, and initiatives that promote physical health contribute to overall employee well-being (Wong et al., 2021). *Crisis management and support:* Being prepared to provide support during times of crisis, such as a pandemic or natural disaster, demonstrates a commitment to employees' safety and well-being (Liu et al., 2020). *Leadership development:* Including empathy training in leadership development programs helps leaders understand and respond to the emotional needs of their teams (Ahmed et al., 2020, Qin & Men, 2023). *Professional growth opportunities:* Providing clear career paths and opportunities for professional development gives employees a sense of purpose and direction, contributing to their overall well-being (Mikołajczyk, 2022).

Employee surveys and feedback: Conducting regular surveys and seeking feedback from employees allows organizations to understand their concerns and make informed decisions to enhance well-being (Qin & Men, 2023). *Financial well-being support:* Offering financial education programs and support services helps employees manage their finances and reduce stress related to financial concerns (Wong et al., 2021). *Community engagement and social impact:* Involving employees in corporate social responsibility (CSR) initiatives and community engagement activities fosters a sense of purpose and community, positively impacting their well-being (Zhang & Wang, 2022). *Technology for well-being:* Leveraging technology, such as well-being apps and platforms, can provide employees with tools and resources to manage stress, practice mindfulness, and maintain a healthy lifestyle (Hai et al., 2021). *Clear expectations and goal setting:* Establishing clear expectations and realistic goals helps employees manage workloads, reduce stress, and enhance overall well-being (Daneshfar et al., 2023). *Periodic well-being check-ins:* Periodic check-ins on employee well-being, either through surveys or one-on-one conversations, help organizations understand evolving needs and tailor support accordingly (Kaushik & Guleria, 2020). Focusing on employee well-being and fostering a culture of empathy would not only improve the health and happiness of the workforce but also raise their productivity, retention, and overall organizational success in the post-COVID-19 landscape.

7.4   Supply chain resilience

The pandemic exposed vulnerabilities in global supply chains with many businesses facing disruptions due to lockdowns, travel restrictions, and shortages of essential materials, which resulted in managers learning the importance of building resilient supply chains that can withstand shocks (Moosavi et al., 2022). Diversifying suppliers, localizing production when possible, and maintaining strategic reserves are strategies that can enhance supply chain resilience (Kazancoglu et al., 2022). In post-COVID-19 economy, supply chain resilience has become a critical focus for businesses as they seek to enhance their ability to adapt to disruptions and build a more robust and agile supply chain (Panwar et al., 2022). In this section, we discuss some key considerations and strategies for supply chain resilience in the post-pandemic era.

Diversification of suppliers to reduce dependency: Businesses need to diversify their supplier base to reduce dependency on a single source to minimize the impact of disruptions caused by events such as natural disasters, geopolitical issues, or global health crises (Kazancoglu et al., 2022). *Regionalization and nearshoring:* Businesses are discovering the advantages of regionalizing their supply chains and relying on nearshoring which involves sourcing from local and regional suppliers that are closer in proximity. All these steps help businesses reduce lead times, transportation costs, and impact of global disruptions on the supply chain (Panwar et al., 2022). *Digitalization and advanced technologies:* Businesses need to integrate emerging technologies (e.g., IoT, AI, and blockchain) to enhance visibility and traceability across the supply chain using real-time data and analytics to monitor the process and respond to potential disruptions promptly (Modgil et al., 2022).

Risk management and scenario planning: Businesses need to conduct risk assessments and implement risk mitigation strategies using tools, such as scenario planning, to help them prepare for potential disruptions and allow for more agile responses (Wang et al., 2023). *Collaboration and stronger partnerships with suppliers:* Building strong relationships with suppliers would foster collaborative spirit and mutual trust to facilitate more open communications and information exchange among partnerships, which in turn can lead to shared risk management strategies and coordinated responses to disruptions (Kwok et al., 2019). *Inventory optimization:* Maintaining optimal inventory levels helps buffer against disruptions and hence, businesses need to use advanced inventory management techniques to avoid excess and obsolete inventory (Ozdemir et al., 2022). *Agile manufacturing processes:* Adopting agile manufacturing processes enables quick adjustments to production schedules based on changes in demand, disruptions, or supply chain dynamics (Panwar et al., 2022).

End-to-end supply chain visibility: Businesses need to enhance visibility across the entire supply chain, including supplier networks, transportation, and inventory levels, to identify potential issues before they escalate (Kazancoglu et al., 2022). *Sustainability and environmental considerations:* Businesses need to integrate sustainable business practices, such as responsible sourcing and ethical considerations, into their supply chain processes as these practices not only contribute to environmental goals but also enhance resilience (Mattera et al., 2021). *Employee training and skill development:* Businesses would find it useful to invest in training and skill development of their employees to ensure that they have the required expertise to effectively manage and optimize the supply chain at all times (Chun et al., 2021). *Data security and cybersecurity:* As supply chains become more digital and data-driven, managers need to ensure that they have robust data security and cybersecurity measures in place, as these are crucial to prevent disruptions caused by cyber threats (Lallie et al., 2021).

Alternative transportation routes and diverse modes: Identifying alternative transportation routes and modes would help businesses navigate disruptions in traditional supply chain routes, such as ports or key transportation corridors (Panwar et al., 2022). ***Business continuity planning:*** Having comprehensive business continuity plans in place would ensure that organizations can quickly resume operations after a disruption, minimizing downtime and financial impact (Margherita & Heikkilä, 2021). ***Adaptability to market changes through demand sensing:*** Businesses need to adopt new technologies to be able to sense market demand in real-time, which would allow them to quickly adjust their production and supply chain strategies based on changing customer preferences and environmental factors that may disrupt supply chains and hurt their regular operations (Singh et al., 2023).

Resilient logistics networks through flexible partnerships: Businesses should aim to have resilient logistics networks and flexible partnerships with logistics providers as it would help them quickly adjust in response to supply chain disruptions (Panwar et al., 2022). ***Regulatory compliance and adaptation:*** Managers should keep informed and compliant with changing regulations to ensure that their supply chains are not disrupted due to legal or compliance issues (Uddin et al., 2023). ***Continuous improvement and learning from disruptions:*** After disruptions, businesses should conduct thorough post-event analyses to identify areas for improvement. Continuous learning and improvement are essential for building long-term resilience (Moosavi et al., 2022; Ozdemir et al., 2022). ***Strategic stockpiling of critical components:*** Businesses would find it useful to stockpile critical components or materials, particularly those with long lead times or limited availability, to buffer against shortages during supply chain disruptions (Sodhi et al., 2023).

Effective crisis communication planning: Businesses should establish clear communication plans for internal and external stakeholders during crises to more effectively manage their expectations and maintain trust in the supply chain (Moosavi et al., 2022). ***Use advanced technologies to improve predictive capabilities:*** Leveraging artificial intelligence (AI) and predictive analytics would enable businesses to anticipate potential disruptions, allowing for proactive risk management and decision-making (Modgil et al., 2022). ***Build resilient supply chain culture:*** Fostering a resilient supply chain culture involves instilling a mindset of adaptability, continuous improvement, and proactive risk management throughout the organization (Ozdemir et al., 2022). Supply chain resilience in the post-COVID-19 era requires a holistic approach that incorporates technological advancements, strategic planning, collaboration, and a commitment to continuous improvement. Businesses that prioritize these elements are better positioned to navigate uncertainties and disruptions in the global supply chain landscape (Kazancoglu et al., 2022; Moosavi et al., 2022; Ozdemir et al., 2022; Panwar et al., 2022).

7.5 Crisis preparedness

The pandemic underscored the necessity of being prepared for unexpected crises. Managers should incorporate scenario planning and risk assessment into their strategic thinking. Preparing for a range of possible disruptions, from health crises to natural disasters, can enable organizations to respond more effectively when such events occur. In post-COVID-19 period, organizations are placing a significant emphasis on crisis preparedness to ensure they are resilient in the face of various challenges. In this section, we describe some important considerations and strategies to help businesses remain prepared to face any major crisis in the post-pandemic era.

Comprehensive risk assessments: Conducting thorough risk assessments would help organizations identify potential threats and vulnerabilities, ranging from natural disasters to economic downturns (Augustin et al., 2022). *Scenario planning and crisis simulation:* Scenario planning involves simulating various crisis situations to prepare for a range of potential disruptions, which helps organizations develop effective response strategies (Moosavi et al., 2022). *Establish crisis response teams:* Having dedicated crisis response teams with defined roles and responsibilities would ensure a coordinated and effective response during a crisis (Liu et al., 2021). *Crisis simulations and drills as regular practice:* Conducting crisis simulations and drills regularly helps organizations test their crisis response plans and identify areas for improvement (Reddin et al., 2021).

Global risk management: For organizations with global operations, understanding and managing geopolitical and global risks are critical components of crisis preparedness (Wang et al., 2023). *Comprehensive insurance policies:* Regularly reviewing and updating insurance coverage ensures that organizations are adequately protected against various types of risks (Bisco et al., 2020). *Third-party risk management:* Evaluating and managing risks associated with third-party vendors and partners ensure the resilience of the entire business ecosystem (Wang et al., 2023). *Regulatory compliance and monitoring:* Regularly monitoring changes in regulations and compliance requirements helps organizations stay aligned with legal standards during and after a crisis (Uddin et al., 2023). *Legal and compliance preparedness:* Staying informed about and compliant with relevant regulations ensures that organizations are not exposed to legal risks during a crisis (Sheldon, 2021).

Technology readiness and infrastructure resilience: Ensuring that technology infrastructure is robust and resilient helps organizations maintain operational continuity during disruptions (Hai et al., 2021). *Data security and privacy measures:* Strengthening data security and privacy measures ensures that organizations can protect sensitive information, especially during cyber crises (Lallie et al., 2021). *Supply chain diversification:* Having diversified supplier networks and creating redundancies in the supply chain minimize the impact of disruptions on the availability of goods and services (Panwar et al., 2022). *Financial resilience*: Maintaining reserves and having contingency plans for financial challenges enhance organizational resilience during economic downturns or unexpected expenses (Margherita & Heikkilä, 2021). *Investment in developing resilience:* Allocating resources to invest in resilience measures, including technology, employee training, and infrastructure, demonstrates a commitment to long-term organizational stability (Mattera et al., 2021).

Employee training and awareness: Providing employees with training on crisis response, including evacuation procedures, first aid, and cybersecurity awareness, prepares them to act effectively during emergencies (Chun et al., 2021). *Flexible remote work policies:* Having established remote work policies allows organizations to quickly implement and adapt to remote work arrangements during crises that require physical distancing (Daneshfar et al., 2023). *Community engagement and CSR:* Organizations embedded in their communities can leverage these relationships during a crisis, receiving support and assistance from local stakeholders (Zhang & Wang, 2022). *Clear communication protocols:* Developing clear communication protocols and plans ensures that information is disseminated effectively to internal and external stakeholders during a crisis (Kharbat et al., 2023). *Media relations strategies and training:* Training spokespersons and having media relations strategies in place help manage the organization's public image during a crisis (Qin & Men, 2023). *Stakeholder engagement:* Building strong relationships and regular communication with key stakeholders to foster trust ensures a more cooperative response during crises (Bullock et al., 2022).

Public health measures and safety protocols: Implementing and communicating health and safety measures, including hygiene protocols, support employee well-being during health-related crises (Liu et al., 2020). *Crisis debriefing and learning:* After a crisis, conducting a thorough debriefing and analysis helps organizations learn from the experience and refine their crisis preparedness plans (Liu et al., 2020). *Adaptive and agile leadership:* Leaders with adaptive skills can guide organizations through crises effectively, making informed decisions and providing steady guidance (Ahmed et al., 2020). *Cross-functional collaborative approach:* Encouraging cross-functional collaboration ensures that different departments work together seamlessly during a crisis, providing a coordinated response (Chesbrough, 2020). *Crisis recovery strategies:* Developing clear recovery plans outline the steps to be taken after the crisis has subsided, facilitating a smoother return to normal operations (Rahman et al., 2021). Overall, crisis preparedness is an ongoing effort that involves continuous improvement and adaptation to face the ever-changing and evolving challenges. Organizations that prioritize a proactive and comprehensive approach to crisis preparedness would be better equipped to navigate uncertainties and emerge stronger from crises in future.

7.6 Clear communication and change management

Clear and transparent communication became a lifeline during the pandemic. Managers learned that providing accurate information to employees, customers, and stakeholders is crucial, even when the situation is uncertain. Timely communication helps build trust and credibility, and it can prevent the spread of misinformation. Clear communication by managers is crucial, especially in the post-COVID-19 era where uncertainties and changes continue to impact workplaces. Effective communication by managers plays a crucial role in fostering trust, collaboration, and a positive work environment. By prioritizing clarity, empathy, and adaptability, managers can navigate the post-COVID-19 landscape and lead their teams effectively through ongoing changes. In this section, we discuss some key issues and suggestions for effective communication by managers during major crises such as the recent pandemic.

Openness and transparency about changes: Businesses need to be transparent about any changes within their organization, whether related to policies, procedures, or the overall business strategy (Minbaeva et al., 2018). Managers should address uncertainties with candid and straightforward communication. *Empathy to understand employee concerns:* Organizations should develop and demonstrate empathy towards their employees by acknowledging the challenges they may be facing, to understand and address their concerns, both professionally and personally (Ahmed et al., 2020). *Clear and concise communication:* Managers should deliver messages in a clear and concise manner, avoiding jargon and ensuring that the information is easily understandable by all employees irrespective of their levels and roles (Kharbat et al., 2023). *Encourage feedback:* Organizations need to foster an environment where employees feel comfortable providing feedback and sharing their knowledge with the management because such two-way communication is essential for a better understanding of employee needs and concerns (Qin & Men, 2023). *Provide easy access to information:* Organizations should ensure that all the important information is easily accessible to all the employees and to achieve this objective, they should use all available communication channels, such as emails, intranet, and team meetings, to share crucial information (Liu et al., 2020).

Adaptable and flexible communication style: Recognize that different situations and employees in different roles and at different levels may require different communication approaches. Hence, managers should adapt their communication style to fit the context and the recipients, for both positive or challenging announcements (Qin & Men, 2023). *Regular updates with consistent communication:* Organizations should provide regular updates on their current status, changes, and future plans to their employees as this would help them build trust and keep their employees informed (Liu et al., 2020). *Effective remote communication:* Organizations should develop effective virtual communication practices for their remote and hybrid teams, using diverse tools including video conferences and collaborative platforms, to maintain contact through regular check-ins (Qin & Men, 2023). *Crisis communication plans:* Managers should develop crisis communication plans and use these when needed, in order to ensure that employees are aware of the steps to take during emergencies or unexpected events (Liu et al., 2020). *Aligning communication with goals:* Managers should ensure that their communications are aligned with the organization's goals by clearly articulating how individual and team efforts contribute to the overall success of the organization (Qin & Men, 2023). *Timely updates:* Timeliness of information is crucial in communication so managers should provide timely updates during periods of change or uncertainty (Liu et al., 2020).

Set clear expectations: Managers should clearly communicate expectations regarding work arrangements, performance standards, and any changes in policies as this would help employees understand their roles and responsibilities, especially during crisis situations (Daneshfar et al., 2023). *Recognize and appreciate contributions:* Organizations should recognize and appreciate the efforts of employees by publicly acknowledging their achievements and contributions, as this would help them boost employee morale and motivation (Wong et al., 2021). *Prioritizing employee well-being:* Managers should consciously include discussions about employee well-being in their communications, ranging from mental health support to a healthy work-life balance, to demonstrate their commitment to employee well-being (Liu et al., 2020). *Effective communication training for managers:* Organizations should not assume their managers to be effective communicators and need to provide appropriate training to them for improving their communication skills, which may include active listening, providing constructive feedback, and fostering open dialogue (Sangster Jokić & Jokić-Begić, 2022).

Cultural sensitivity: In diverse workplaces, managers should always be mindful of cultural differences in communication styles to ensure that their messages are inclusive and sensitive to diverse cultural perspectives held by their employees (Colleoni et al., 2022). *Personalized communication:* Whenever possible, managers may personalize their communication by addressing individuals by name or tailoring messages to specific teams or departments to make these more directly relevant (Wetherall et al., 2022). *Address concerns proactively:* Managers should not simply wait for bad news to trickle back to them, instead, they should anticipate tough questions and concerns about the organization's policies and actions in a proactive manner. (Wang et al., 2023). This would help them prevent any misinformation or confusion by directly addressing any potential questions or concerns that employees might have. *Fostering collaborative communication:* Organizations need to encourage collaboration among teams by facilitating open communication channels using platforms for team discussions and idea sharing to contribute to a collaborative environment (Bernardo et al., 2021). *Learn from feedback:* Organizations should establish a feedback loop that makes employees feel comfortable enough to provide feedback on its policies and practices. Managers should then use this feedback to continuously improve their communication strategies (Sangster Jokić & Jokić-Begić, 2022).

Cultivate and promote positive culture: Managers should use their communication to cultivate a positive organizational culture by emphasizing shared values, goals, and collective effort toward success (Colleoni et al., 2022). *Celebrate achievements and highlight successes:* Organizations should celebrate team and individual achievements with positive communication about successes that contribute to a positive and motivated workplace (Qin & Men, 2023). ***Manage workplace changes:*** Managers should recognize and address the unique challenges faced by their employees, such as potential feelings of isolation caused by remote working arrangements, and they should facilitate open communications with the employees to alleviate their concerns on such issues (Yue & Walden, 2023). ***Prepare employees for future changes:*** Organizations need to communicate any anticipated changes in advance to prepare their employees for future adjustments that they may need to make. Such transparency would help them in managing employee expectations (Yue & Walden, 2023).

7.7 Global interconnectedness

As the pandemic highlighted the interconnected nature of our world, managers understood that local actions can have global ramifications, and this realization underscored the need to consider the broader social and environmental impact of their decisions (Bernardo et al., 2021). The pandemic had profound effects on global interconnectedness, influencing various aspects of international relations, trade, and collaboration which are going to become even more important in the post-COVID era with a complex interplay of challenges and opportunities. Countries, businesses, and organizations would need to navigate this landscape by fostering cooperation, leveraging technology, and adapting to new norms to address shared global concerns. In this section, we discuss the importance of understanding current trends in global interconnectedness and their implications for businesses and managers in the post-COVID-19 era.

Reshape international relations with shifts in global alliances: The pandemic prompted shifts in international relations and alliances as countries reassessed their geopolitical and economic partnerships. Hence, individual countries and businesses need to reprioritize their international alliances to take into account these changes (Bernardo et al., 2021). ***Accelerated digital transformation with greater digital connectivity:*** The pandemic accelerated digital transformation, leading to increased reliance on digital technologies for communication, commerce, and collaboration on a global scale, which has significant implications for multinational companies aspiring to grow their businesses globally (Hai et al., 2021). ***Reevaluate global supply chains:*** Businesses and countries are reevaluating and restructuring their supply chains to enhance resilience, including considerations for local sourcing and reducing dependencies on specific regions (Panwar et al., 2022). ***Global workforce connectivity through remote work and collaboration:*** Remote work has become more prevalent, enabling professionals to collaborate across borders seamlessly, which has implications for talent acquisition, diversity, and collaboration (Jones et al., 2023). ***International travel challenges:*** The pandemic has significantly impacted international travel, affecting tourism and business travel, with the industry being forced to adapt to new norms and regulations (Stobart & Duckett, 2022).

Public health diplomacy through global health cooperation: The pandemic highlighted the importance of global health cooperation. Countries are likely to focus on strengthening international mechanisms for pandemic preparedness and response (Liu et al., 2020). *Digital platforms for diplomacy:* During and after the pandemic, diplomats and leaders increasingly used digital platforms for diplomatic engagements and international cooperation, influencing the nature of global diplomacy (Hai et al., 2021). *Interconnectedness in global economic recovery:* The global economy's recovery is interconnected with the economic health of one region influencing others. Hence, global cooperation is essential for sustainable recovery (Bernardo et al., 2021). *Collaboration in scientific research:* The pandemic emphasized the importance of international collaboration in scientific research and knowledge-sharing, influencing future research and development efforts (Bernardo et al., 2021). *Technological interdependence:* The technology sector is globally interconnected, with innovations, disruptions, and cybersecurity concerns impacting countries and industries worldwide (Liu et al., 2020).

Global efforts for climate change: International cooperation on addressing climate change is crucial for a sustainable future, wherein countries are expected to collaborate on climate policies and initiatives (Klenert et al., 2020). *Expansion of cross-border e-commerce:* E-commerce has become a significant driver of global trade and its growth is reshaping how businesses engage with their customers and competitors in the international markets (Karpen et al., 2020). *Calls for international governance reforms:* The pandemic has prompted discussions about reforming international governance structures to better address global challenges and ensure equitable distribution of resources (Liu et al., 2021). *Global talent mobility:* Remote work and online education have increased global talent mobility, allowing individuals to contribute to projects and organizations regardless of geographic location (Vaiman et al., 2021). *Shifts in migration patterns:* The pandemic has also influenced migration trends, impacting workforce demographics and contributing to discussions about immigration policies related to global education and skill mobility (Sirkeci & Yüceşahin, 2020). *Global academic partnerships:* Higher education institutions such as universities and research institutions are expanding international collaborations in education and research to address global challenges (Kong & Wu, 2023).

Health diplomacy (International collaboration in healthcare): Health diplomacy is gaining prominence as countries collaborate on healthcare initiatives, research, and sharing best practices (Liu et al., 2020). *Vaccine diplomacy in global vaccine distribution:* The distribution of vaccines globally highlights the concept of vaccine diplomacy, where countries engage in diplomatic efforts through vaccine donations and collaborations (Sparke & Levy, 2022). *Humanitarian and development assistance (Global aid and assistance):* The interconnectedness of global challenges has underscored the importance of international cooperation in providing humanitarian and development assistance (Gazi & Gazis, 2020). *Global diversity, equity, and inclusion (DEI) initiatives:* There is an increasing focus on global diversity, equity, and inclusion initiatives as organizations recognize the importance of diverse perspectives in a connected world (Jones et al., 2023).

   Global cybersecurity cooperation: The interconnectedness of digital systems requires global collaboration to address cybersecurity threats effectively (Lallie et al., 2021). *Social and cultural exchange:* Social and cultural exchanges have adapted to digital platforms, allowing for continued global interactions despite travel restrictions (Colleoni et al., 2022). *Reevaluate post-pandemic international trade policies:* Countries are reevaluating their trade policies in the post-pandemic era, considering factors such as supply chain resilience, protectionism, and fair trade practices (Sharma et al., 2020). *Global data governance:* The cross-border flow of data and privacy concerns are driving discussions on global data governance frameworks (Lallie et al., 2021). *Crisis response preparedness and cooperation:* The interconnected nature of global challenges emphasizes the need for international preparedness and cooperation in responding to crises (Liu et al., 2020).

7.8   Continuous learning and upskilling

The rapidly changing landscape during the pandemic emphasized the importance of continuous learning and upskilling with managers recognizing that staying updated with industry trends and acquiring new skills is essential for personal and organizational growth (Falkner et al., 2022). This experience has highlighted the value of investing in employee development. Continuous learning and upskilling have become increasingly critical in the post-COVID-19 era as industries evolve, technology advances, and new skills become essential (Hai et al., 2021). Continuous learning and upskilling are integral to staying competitive in today's dynamic and evolving professional landscape. By actively seeking new knowledge, adapting to industry changes, and fostering a mindset of growth, individuals can position themselves for success in the post-COVID-19 era. In this section, we discuss the importance and implications of continuous learning and upskilling for both individuals and organizations in the post-COVID-19 era.

   Adapting to digital transformation: Embrace digital literacy by learning and mastering essential digital tools and technologies. This is crucial as organizations increasingly rely on digital platforms and remote work (Hai et al., 2021). *Effective remote collaboration:* Develop skills that support effective remote collaboration, including virtual communication, project management tools, and online collaboration platforms (Daneshfar et al., 2023). *Technical skills and proficiency:* Managers need to stay updated on relevant technologies in their industry to upskill in areas like data analytics, AI, and cybersecurity can enhance their career prospects (Falkner et al., 2022). *Soft skills development:* Focus on developing soft skills, including emotional intelligence, adaptability, and effective communication. These skills are crucial for navigating diverse work environments. *Agile and critical thinking:* Cultivate agile thinking and critical problem-solving skills. The ability to adapt to changing circumstances and analyze complex situations is highly valued (Ozdemir et al., 2022; Panwar et al., 2022).

Industry-specific training: Organizations should offer industry-specific training and certifications to their managers and employees to help them stay current with trends, regulations, and best practices within their fields (Sangster Jokić & Jokić-Begić, 2022). *Lifelong learning mindset to build curiosity and openness:* Managers should cultivate a mindset of lifelong learning. Stay curious, open to new ideas, and actively seek opportunities for personal and professional growth (Çelik et al., 2023). *Cross-functional skills and knowledge:* Organizations should help their employees develop cross-functional skills that span multiple disciplines to make them more adaptable and valuable in various roles (Chesbrough, 2020). *Professional networking and mentoring:* Engage in professional networking to learn from others in your industry. Seek out mentors who can provide guidance and share their experiences (Wong et al., 2021). *Microlearning:* Embrace microlearning, which involves short, targeted learning sessions. This approach allows for continuous learning without significant time commitments.

Cultural awareness and competence: Develop cultural competence to work effectively with diverse teams and navigate global business environments (Papadopoulos, 2022). *Cross-cultural communication skills:* Develop cross-cultural communication skills to effectively interact with colleagues, clients, and partners from diverse cultural backgrounds (Chae et al., 2023). *Language and communication skills:* Enhance language skills, particularly for employees working in an international context as effective communication is crucial in diverse and global workplaces (Sangster Jokić & Jokić-Begić, 2022). *Entrepreneurial skills:* Foster an entrepreneurial mindset, even within larger organizations. This involves taking initiative, being innovative, and embracing a proactive approach (Wardana et al., 2023). *Project management skills:* Consider obtaining a project management certification to enhance your ability to plan, execute, and oversee projects effectively (Marhraoui, 2023). *E-learning trends:* Keep yourself informed about emerging trends in e-learning, including new technologies, methodologies, and platforms that enhance the learning experience (Adedoyin & Soykan, 2023). *Online learning platforms and courses:* Leverage online learning platforms offering courses and certifications in various subjects. Platforms like Coursera, LinkedIn Learning, and edX provide access to a wide range of courses (García-Morales et al., 2021).

Continuous feedback: Organizations should establish a culture of continuous feedback to allow employees to seek feedback on their performance and provide constructive feedback to their colleagues (Qin & Men, 2023). *Professional development planning:* Managers should create and follow individual development plans to outline their career goals, identify necessary skills, and map out steps to achieve them (Mikołajczyk, 2022). *Industry conferences and events:* Managers should attend industry conferences, webinars, and events to stay updated on the latest developments, connect with professionals, and gain insights. ***Regular self-assessment:*** Managers should regularly assess their skills and identify areas that require improvement as this self-awareness is key to planning effective upskilling efforts. ***Leadership development and training:*** For employees aspiring to leadership roles, organizations should invest in leadership development programs to enhance their strategic thinking, decision-making, and team management skills. ***Evolving industry trends analysis:*** Managers should stay informed about evolving industry trends to anticipate future skill requirements and proactively acquire the skills that will be in demand. ***Collaborative and team-based learning:*** Organizations should embrace collaborative learning within teams to encourage knowledge-sharing, peer-to-peer learning, and collaborative problem-solving (Bernardo et al., 2021). ***Flexible learning models to balance work and learning:*** Managers may explore flexible learning models that allow them to balance work commitments with ongoing learning, including part-time courses or evening classes (Tulaskar & Turunen, 2022).

7.9   Conclusion

COVID-19 has been a powerful teacher for managers across the globe teaching us lessons that go beyond crisis management and offer insights into adaptability, empathy, technological readiness, and more. As the world moves forward, integrating these lessons into managerial practices can pave the way for more resilient, innovative, and compassionate organizations and help them develop suitable strategies to face such crises in future. For example, we have learned that the ability to adapt quickly to unforeseen circumstances is crucial in managing any unexpected crisis. Hence, businesses should build a culture of resilience and flexibility to navigate uncertainties. We also saw that companies with robust digital infrastructure fared better than others. Hence, businesses should accelerate their digital transformation efforts to improve their agility and efficiency. Similarly, we have seen that remote work is viable and can enhance productivity and reduce costs. Hence, more businesses should embrace hybrid work models and invest in collaboration tools for remote and in-office teams, as far as possible.

One of the critical challenges during COVID-19 was managing supply chain disruptions due to over-reliance on specific suppliers from certain regions (e.g., China). To address this issue, businesses should diversify their supply chains and establish contingency plans for better risk management. Another key issue was the retention of customers for business survival especially as many businesses could not rely on their traditional models with rapid changes in customer needs and preferences. Hence, businesses would find it useful to prioritize customer experience, leverage data for insights, and personalize offerings. At the same time, we also learned the importance of maintaining strong financial reserves to weather unexpected crises, and therefore, businesses should adopt conservative financial practices and stress-test their business and funding models regularly to avoid any unpleasant surprises.

On a more positive note, we saw e-commerce platforms and businesses gain prominence during lockdowns, which offers an opportunity for more businesses to strengthen their online presence and develop omni-channel strategies to meet diverse customer preferences. Another silver lining to the dark cloud of the pandemic was the realization of the importance of employee well-being for business continuity. We hope this will encourage more businesses to prioritize health and safety measures in their workplaces, especially as new threats emerge. Similarly, businesses are now increasingly expected to contribute to social and environmental goals by integrating these goals into their business strategies for long-term success. We also learned that global challenges require international cooperation, which highlights the need to collaborate with global partners, governments, and organizations to address shared challenges.

Finally, we saw that quick decision-making was vital for the survival of businesses during the pandemic, which should encourage more businesses to foster a culture of agile decision-making and empower teams to act swiftly. To conclude, businesses should learn from the adaptability demonstrated during the pandemic, prioritize digital transformation, focus on customer needs, diversify supply chains, and foster a resilient and socially responsible organizational culture. The future outlook emphasizes ongoing evolution, with a particular focus on technology, employee well-being, and sustainable business practices, to face any unanticipated crisis in the post-pandemic era.

8 Conclusion and recommendations

8.1 Conduct comprehensive risk assessments

Conducting a comprehensive risk assessment involves identifying, analyzing, and evaluating potential risks that could affect an organization. Regular assessment of potential risks to any business, both internal and external, may include financial risks, supply chain vulnerabilities, and market-specific threats. Managers should consider a wide range of scenarios, from natural disasters to economic downturns, and pandemics, to develop their response plans. Overall, conducting a comprehensive risk assessment is an ongoing process that requires commitment, collaboration, and adaptability. By systematically identifying, analyzing, and mitigating risks, organizations can enhance their resilience and make informed decisions to achieve their objectives, which is going to be extremely important in the post-COVID-19 era. We recommend the following step-by-step guide to conducting a thorough risk assessment:

Establish the context: Managers should begin by clearly defining the scope and objectives of the risk assessment, which would involve identifying the assets, processes, and activities that will be assessed. This can be done by creating an inventory of the organization's assets, including physical assets, intellectual property, data, personnel, and key processes.

Risk identification: The next step would be to conduct brainstorming sessions with relevant stakeholders to identify potential risks, which would help consider internal and external factors that could impact the organization. Once the managers have identified risks, these should be classified into categories, such as financial, operational, strategic, compliance, and reputational, to help them organize and prioritize different types of risks.

Risk analysis: Next, the managers should qualitatively assess the extent and likelihood of the impact of each identified risk, using a risk matrix to categorize risks based on their severity and probability. This could be followed with a quantitative assessment (if possible) by assigning monetary values to the different types of risks for a numerical analysis, which would help estimate the potential financial losses associated with each type of risk.

Risk prioritization: The next step would involve prioritization of risks based on their severity and potential impact on the organization, to help the

DOI: 10.4324/9781003227113-9

organization's focus on high-priority risks that may require immediate attention. This process also involves defining the organization's risk tolerance level to help the managers understand the level of risk their organization is willing to accept or mitigate during any unexpected situation.

Control assessment: Managers should also identify and assess existing controls and mitigation measures in place for each identified risk, to evaluate their effectiveness in reducing or eliminating the risk. Using a gap analysis can also help the managers identify areas where existing controls are insufficient or ineffective, which in turn would guide them to develop additional controls, as and when required.

Risk mitigation: Managers should develop hypothetical scenarios for high-impact risks to help them understand their potential cascading effects and prepare response plans. For example, they may use the findings from their risk analysis, to develop specific mitigation strategies for each high-priority risk, which may include implementing new controls, transferring risk, or avoiding certain activities.

Risk management: Risk management is an ongoing exercise and to do this, organizations should establish a system for continuous monitoring and review of all the different types of risks. Regular review and update of the risk assessment would reflect the changes in the organization's environment and help respond to these changes in a proactive manner.

Risk communication: Managers should communicate the results of their risk assessment to the relevant stakeholders in a timely and regular manner, to ensure that key decision-makers are aware of the identified risks and mitigation strategies. Comprehensive documentation of the entire risk assessment process, including the identified risks, analysis methods, and mitigation plans, is crucial for future reference and audits.

Risk response: Organizations should provide relevant training to their employees on risk awareness and the importance of adhering to risk mitigation measures as a well-informed workforce contributes to a more resilient and responsive organization. Managers should also ensure that the entire risk assessment process aligns with relevant industry regulations and compliance requirements, which is particularly important for heavily regulated industries.

Risk embeddedness: Managers should aim to integrate their risk management strategies into the organization's daily operations and decision-making processes, to ensure that risk considerations are part of strategic planning and execution. To achieve this objective, it is crucial for them to encourage feedback from stakeholders involved in the risk assessment process. Use this feedback to continuously improve the risk management framework.

Risk responsiveness: Managers should take into account external factors, such as economic conditions, geopolitical events, and industry trends, which may all impact their organization's risk landscape. To achieve this objective, managers should recognize that the risk landscape is dynamic in nature, and managing risk requires regular reassessment of risks and updating mitigation strategies to be able to adapt to changes in the internal and external environment.

Risk culture: Organizations should aim to foster a culture that encourages employees to be aware of and proactively address risks, by promoting open communication about potential risks. In some complex scenarios, managers may consider seeking the expertise of external consultants or specialists to ensure a comprehensive and unbiased risk assessment.

Risk leadership and planning: Managers should involve board members and organizational leaders in the risk assessment process, as their engagement is crucial to set risk management priorities and ensure organizational alignment and commitment. To achieve this objective, they would need to integrate the risk assessment outcomes into the organization's crisis response plans to ensure a coordinated and informed approach during crises.

8.2 Develop a crisis response plan

One of the key learnings from the pandemic has been the need to create a detailed crisis response plan that outlines roles, responsibilities, and decision-making processes during a crisis. Such a plan should also include communication protocols for employees, customers, suppliers, and other stakeholders. Organizations may also designate a crisis management team with clear leadership roles to develop a crisis response plan, which is crucial for them to effectively navigate and manage unexpected events. Developing a crisis response plan is an ongoing process that requires regular updates and testing. The plan should be dynamic, adaptable to different scenarios, and reflective of the organization's commitment to the safety and well-being of its employees and stakeholders. Regular reviews, training sessions, and drills will contribute to the plan's effectiveness in times of unexpected crises. In this section, we provide a step-by-step guide to help managers develop, implement, monitor, and modify a comprehensive crisis response plan.

Establish a crisis management team: The first step towards developing a crisis response plan is to form a crisis management team, which should consist of key personnel from various departments, including people with expertise in communication, operations, legal, human resources, and other relevant areas.

Risk assessment: Managers should conduct a thorough risk assessment to identify potential crises that could impact the organization, including any possible internal and external factors that may pose a threat to the organization and its normal operations.

Define objectives and scope: Next, the managers should define the objectives of the crisis response plan, which would help them clearly specify the scope of the plan, identify the types of crises it will address, and the geographical areas covered.

Establish communication protocols: This step involves defining clear communication protocols for internal and external stakeholders, by specifying who communicates what information, through which channels, and at what intervals.

Establish chain of command: Organizations should clearly outline the chain of command during a crisis, which would involve identifying the key decision-makers and establishing a hierarchy to ensure efficient communication and well-informed decision-making.

Emergency contact information: Organizations should also compile and maintain an updated list of emergency contact information for all crisis management team members, key personnel, and relevant external contacts at all times to avoid any unexpected surprises.

Crisis response plan documentation: Managers should document the crisis response plan in a comprehensive written document, which may include all essential information, procedures, and contact details, needed to effectively handle any crisis situation.

Conduct training sessions: Organizations should train the crisis management team and relevant employees on the crisis response plan by conducting regular drills and simulations to ensure everyone is familiar with their roles and responsibilities and ready to deliver the same.

Identify resources: Managers should identify the resources required to implement the crisis response plan, which may include personnel, technology, equipment, and any external support needed to respond successfully to any unexpected crisis.

Establish response procedures: Managers should also develop detailed response procedures for each type of crisis identified in the risk assessment by clearly outlining the steps to be taken during the initial response and subsequent phases.

Develop evacuation and shelter plans: Organizations should also create evacuation and shelter plans (if required) to ensure that employees and visitors are familiar at all times with the evacuation routes and designated safe areas, in case these are needed in any emergency.

Develop media relations protocols: Organizations should establish a media relations strategy by designating official spokesperson(s), defining their message strategy, and outlining the procedures for interacting with the media during a crisis.

Consider legal implications: Organizations should also address all possible legal considerations associated with different crises to ensure compliance with all the relevant regulations and legal obligations in their crisis response.

Develop post-crisis recovery plans: Managers should also identify all the steps to be taken to ensure business continuity, reputation management, and returning to normal operations, during and after any unexpected crisis.

Establish external partnerships: Managers should also identify all those external organizations and agencies that can provide support to their organization during a crisis. They should establish partnerships and agreements with these entities well in advance.

Continuous improvement: Organizations should establish a process to collect feedback and conduct a thorough evaluation after each crisis response to identify areas for improvement and update their crisis response plans accordingly.

Ensure regulatory compliance: Organizations should ensure that their crisis response plans are aligned with the relevant regulations and compliance requirements in their industry and appropriate geographical location and jurisdiction.

Communicate with employees: Managers should also develop specific strategies to communicate with their employees during any crisis, to keep them informed about the situation, actions being taken, and any changes to normal operations, which would keep their morale up.

Data protection and privacy: Organizations should develop and implement measures to protect sensitive information during a crisis, which in turn should adhere to the relevant data protection and privacy regulations in the appropriate jurisdiction.

Community engagement: Organizations should develop clear plans to engage with their communities during and after a crisis, to ensure prompt and transparent communication, which would demonstrate their commitment to supporting the community.

Crisis recovery teams: Depending on the nature of the crisis, organizations should form specialized recovery teams, such as IT recovery, supply chain recovery, or financial recovery teams, which may possess the necessary knowledge and skills to address the specific crisis.

Psychological support: Managers should provide psychological support to their employees to address the subjective well-being of employees affected by the crisis. To do this, they would need to establish clear protocols to provide support and mental health resources.

Consider global impact: If the organization operates globally, managers should consider the potential global impacts of any crises faced by their organization, to ensure that their crisis response plans take different cultural and regulatory contexts into account.

Integrate with other plans: Ensure that the crisis response plan is integrated with other organizational plans, such as business continuity plans (BCPs) and disaster recovery plans.

Accessible documentation: Store the crisis response plan in a secure yet accessible location. Ensure that key personnel can access the plan quickly during a crisis.

8.3   Plan and invest in digital transformation

Organizations need to embrace digital transformation to enhance their agility and resilience, using digital communication tools, e-commerce capabilities, and cloud-based systems that allow for remote work and collaboration. At the same time, they also need to develop a robust cybersecurity strategy to protect against cyber threats, which often increase during crises. Planning and investing in digital transformation in post-COVID-19 period requires a strategic and comprehensive approach. We must always remember that digital transformation is an ongoing process, and staying nimble and adaptable is key to long-term success. Hence, managers should regularly reassess their digital transformation strategy to ensure it aligns with the evolving business needs and technological advancements. In this section, we provide a step-by-step guide to help managers navigate this process.

Assess current technologies: Evaluate the existing digital infrastructure, systems, and processes. Evaluate the digital literacy and readiness of the workforce. Clearly define how digital transformation supports the overall business strategy. Establish measurable objectives to track progress.

Engage stakeholders: Involve representatives from IT, operations, marketing, finance, and other relevant departments to create cross-functional teams. Develop a communication plan to keep all stakeholders informed.

Allocate budget and resources: Determine the financial resources required for the digital transformation initiative. Ensure there is a team of right talent or plan for training existing staff. Start with projects that can deliver immediate benefits to build momentum. Prioritize systems critical to the business operations.

Technology selection and evaluation: Research and choose technologies that align with the goals. Consider solutions that can scale with the business growth. Implement robust security measures to protect sensitive data. Ensure that the digital transformation adheres to industry regulations. Equip the workforce with the skills needed for the new digital environment.

Change management: Develop a change management plan to ease the transition. Implement pilot programs to test and refine digital solutions. Roll out digital initiatives in phases. Collect feedback from users to make necessary adjustments. Continuously monitor performance and make adjustments as needed. Regularly evaluate key performance indicators (KPIs). Identify areas for improvement and refine the digital strategy.

Industry collaboration and network: Stay informed about industry trends and collaborate with peers. Explore potential partnerships that can enhance the digital capabilities.

Enhance customer experience: Leverage digital tools to improve customer experience. Establish mechanisms for gathering and acting on customer feedback.

Develop innovation culture: Foster a culture of innovation within the organization. Embrace an agile and adaptable mindset to respond to changing circumstances and be flexible to adjust strategies based on market trends. Conduct regular reviews of the digital transformation strategy.

8.4   Build resilient supply chains

Businesses need to diversify their supply chains to reduce dependencies on a single source or region by having multiple suppliers for critical components, establishing relationships with local suppliers, and considering inshoring or nearshoring key production processes. Building supply chain resilience in post-COVID-19 period is critical for businesses to navigate uncertainties and disruptions. By taking a holistic approach to supply chain resilience, businesses can better prepare for and respond to disruptions, ensuring continuity and adaptability in a rapidly changing environment. Managers should regularly reassess and update their supply chain strategies to stay ahead of emerging challenges. In this section, we describe a few specific steps to help enhance the resilience of supply chains.

Diversify suppliers: Identify and engage with multiple suppliers for critical components or materials. Diversify sources globally and locally to mitigate risks associated with specific regions.

Risk assessment: Conduct a thorough risk assessment to identify vulnerabilities in the supply chain. Prioritize risks based on their potential impact on the operations.

Collaborative relationships through open communication: Foster transparent and open communication with suppliers, customers, and other stakeholders. Develop strategic partnerships with key suppliers for better collaboration during disruptions.

Inventory optimization with buffer stocks: Maintain strategically buffer stock to absorb fluctuations in demand or supply. Modify Just-in-Time (JIT) inventory management systems to allow for more flexibility in supplies.

Technology integration using digital platforms: Utilize digital technologies for real-time visibility into the supply chain. Integrate automation to streamline processes and reduce manual dependencies.

End-to-end supply chain visibility: Implement systems that provide end-to-end visibility into the supply chain. Leverage data analytics to predict and respond to disruptions proactively.

Resilient logistics: Identify alternative transport modes to overcome disruptions in traditional logistics channels. Plan redundant routes for critical shipments.

Scenario planning for contingencies: Develop contingency plans for various disruption scenarios. Conduct desktop exercises and simulations to test the effectiveness of plans.

Regulatory compliance: Understand and comply with regulations affecting the supply chain. Assess and mitigate risks related to geopolitical changes and trade regulations.

Supplier audits and certification: Regularly audit and assess the capabilities and risks associated with the suppliers. Encourage suppliers to adhere to recognized quality and resilience standards.

Employee education and training: Cross-train employees to perform multiple roles to ensure continuity during workforce disruptions. Educate employees on the importance of supply chain resilience.

Insurance and contingency funds: Evaluate insurance options that cover supply chain disruptions. Maintain contingency funds for quick response to unforeseen challenges.

Continuous improvement through feedback mechanisms: Establish feedback loops to continuously improve the supply chain resilience. Be willing to adapt the strategies based on lessons learned from disruptions.

Environmentally sustainable business practices: Integrate sustainable practices into the supply chain for long-term resilience as these may contribute to better risk management.

Legal preparedness through agreements: Ensure that contracts and agreements with suppliers include provisions for force majeure and other unforeseen events. Seek legal advice to understand and mitigate legal risks associated with supply chain disruptions.

8.5   Build and strengthen financial resilience

Businesses need to maintain adequate cash reserves to cover essential operating expenses during any major crisis like the COVID-19 pandemic. They should explore financial instruments like insurance, credit lines, or contingency funds that can provide them with a financial buffer in times of need. Ensuring financial resilience is crucial for the long-term stability and success of a business. By implementing these strategies, businesses can enhance their financial resilience, making them better equipped to withstand economic downturns and unforeseen challenges. Managers need to regularly review and adjust these strategies as their businesses evolve and the economic landscape changes. In this section, we describe a few key strategies that may help managers enhance the financial resilience of their businesses.

Diversify revenue streams with multiple products/services: Offer a range of products or services to diversify income sources. Expand the customer base by targeting diverse markets.

Emergency fund: Build cash reserves. Establish and maintain an emergency fund to cover unexpected expenses. Monitor and manage liquidity to ensure there is cash when needed.

Regular cost reviews: Regularly review and optimize operating costs. Strive to have a higher proportion of variable costs to make it easier to adjust to changing circumstances.

Financial planning and budgeting: Develop and adhere to a comprehensive budget. Implement robust financial forecasting to anticipate potential challenges.

Debt management with prudent borrowing: Be cautious about taking on debt and ensure it aligns with the business strategy. Explore opportunities to refinance debt for better terms.

Comprehensive insurance coverage: Ensure the business has adequate insurance coverage for various risks. Regularly review insurance policies to ensure they remain relevant.

Customer relationship management: Focus on building long-term customer relationships to ensure a steady revenue stream. Avoid dependency on a small number of clients by diversifying the customer base.

Use market research to develop strategy: Keep abreast of industry trends and market changes. Be prepared to adapt the products/services based on market demands.

Efficiency through technology adoption and automation: Utilize technology to improve operational efficiency. Implement automation to reduce manual labor costs.

Employee training and retention: Invest in training. Enhance the skills of the workforce to improve productivity. Retain key talent to avoid recruitment and training costs.

Legal compliance: Adhere to all relevant laws and regulations to avoid legal issues. Periodically review contracts and agreements to ensure compliance and mitigate legal risks.

Strategic partnerships: Collaborate with strategic partners for mutual benefit and form strategic partnerships to share resources and mitigate risks. Work closely with suppliers to negotiate favorable terms.

Continuous monitoring: Conduct regular financial health checks to monitor key financial metrics. Develop and update scenarios for potential economic downturns or disruptions.

Investment in innovation: Adapt to change and invest in innovation to stay relevant in a dynamic business environment. Allocate resources for research and development.

Regulatory compliance and tax planning: Implement effective tax planning strategies to optimize the financial position. Conduct regular internal audits to ensure compliance with regulations.

8.6   Develop employee well-being programs

In the post-pandemic times, businesses need to implement programs that support their employee well-being, both physical and mental, by providing flexible work arrangements, access to mental health resources, and a supportive workplace culture. They can also cross-train employees to ensure flexibility to handle workforce disruptions. Developing employee well-being programs post-COVID-19 period is crucial for maintaining a healthy and engaged workforce. By integrating these strategies into the well-being programs, managers can create a comprehensive approach to address the diverse needs of their workforce in the post-COVID-19 era. Managers also need to regularly assess the impact of these programs and adapt them based on employee feedback and changing circumstances. In this section, we provide a step-by-step guide to help managers create effective employee well-being initiatives for their businesses.

Offer hybrid work models with flexible work arrangements: Implement hybrid work models that balance in-office and remote work. Offer remote work or flexible scheduling to more employees without compromising on the continuity of business operations, if feasible.

Employee assistance programs (EAPs): Provide access to counseling services through EAPs. Provide mental health assistance and encourage the employees to use these services. Offer workshops on building resilience and managing stress through mindfulness sessions and well-being workshops.

Health and fitness programs: Provide subsidies for gym memberships or fitness classes. Organize friendly wellness challenges to encourage physical activity. Organize on-site or virtual health screenings. Offer health risk assessments for employees to identify potential health concerns. Offer resources on healthy eating habits. Provide healthy food and snacks in staff canteen and catering services for events and functions.

Promote a positive work culture: Foster a workplace culture that values positivity and support. Leaders should set an example by prioritizing their well-being. Organize team-building events and activities. Facilitate virtual social interactions for remote or hybrid teams. Establish a system for regular recognition of employee efforts. Encourage peer-to-peer recognition within teams.

Work-life balance: Encourage employees to set clear boundaries between work and personal life. Provide flexibility in work hours to accommodate personal needs. Offer seminars or resources on financial literacy. Help employees understand and optimize their benefits packages. Implement training programs to promote diversity and inclusion. Establish clear policies against discrimination and bias.

Conduct employee surveys: Understand the specific well-being needs and concerns of the employees. Ensure survey responses can be provided anonymously to encourage honest feedback. Ensure that leadership actively supports and participates in well-being programs. Communicate the importance of employee well-being from the top down.

Feedback mechanisms: Regularly gather feedback on well-being programs. Use feedback to adapt and improve initiatives. Define KPIs to measure the impact of well-being programs. Continuously assess the effectiveness of the initiatives.

Communication strategy: Keep employees informed about well-being initiatives. Establish open channels for employees to provide feedback on the programs. Ensure that well-being programs comply with relevant employment laws. Safeguard employee privacy when collecting health-related data.

8.7   Foster a culture of innovation

Managers should encourage innovation within their organization by developing a culture where employees feel empowered to suggest creative solutions during times of crisis. To achieve this objective, they would need to establish processes for rapid decision-making and implementation of innovative ideas. Fostering a culture of innovation is essential for organizations looking to thrive in the post-COVID-19 landscape. By integrating these strategies into their organizational culture, managers can create an environment that not only welcomes innovation but actively nurtures and supports it. Consistent effort and commitment from leadership are crucial to sustaining a culture of innovation over the long term. In this section, we describe a few strategies to encourage innovation within the workplace.

Leadership support: Set the example. Leaders should actively demonstrate and support innovation. Clearly communicate the organization's vision for the future.

Encourage risk-taking: Encourage calculated risk-taking and accept the possibility of failure. Give employees the autonomy to explore and implement their ideas.

Cross-functional collaboration to break down silos: Foster collaboration across departments to break down silos. Form diverse teams with varied skills and perspectives.

Encourage open communication through feedback channels: Establish open channels for employees to share ideas and provide feedback. Create a culture where leaders actively listen to and consider employee input.

Continuous training and skill development: Conduct workshops and training sessions on innovation techniques. Encourage a culture of continuous learning to motivate employees and managers to stay updated on industry trends.

Recognition and rewards: Recognize and reward employees for innovative contributions. Offer incentives such as bonuses or promotions for successful innovations.

Learn from failures: Create an environment where failures are seen as opportunities to learn and improve. Conduct post-mortem analyses to extract lessons from failed projects.

Foster a culture of innovation: Create physical or virtual spaces dedicated to innovation and creative thinking. Ensure these spaces are equipped with tools and resources to support innovation. Align innovation initiatives with overall business goals. Allow dedicated time for employees to work on innovative projects.

Accelerate technology adoption: Embrace new technologies that can enhance innovation processes. Adopt digital collaboration tools to facilitate virtual collaboration and idea sharing.

Develop competitive spirit: Organize regular innovation challenges or hackathons. Encourage employees from different departments to collaborate on solving challenges.

Measure innovation through well-defined metrics: Establish KPIs to measure innovation success. Regularly assess and adjust innovation metrics to ensure their relevance and effectiveness, as needed.

Reward and mentor innovators: Identify and empower innovation champions within the organization. Encourage experienced innovators to mentor others.

Continuous improvement: Promote iterative processes that allow for continuous improvement. Be willing to adapt innovation strategies based on feedback and outcomes.

Customer-centric innovation: Foster a deep understanding of customer needs and preferences. Integrate customer feedback into the innovation process.

Legal considerations to protect intellectual property rights (IPRs): Ensure that processes are in place to protect intellectual property resulting from innovative efforts. Align innovation activities with legal and regulatory requirements.

Share and celebrate successes: Communicate success stories to inspire and motivate employees. Celebrate milestones and achievements related to innovative projects.

Regular reviews and reflections: Regularly review the effectiveness of innovation initiatives. Use reviews to learn from experiences and adjust innovation strategies.

8.8   Crisis management and communication protocols

Businesses should have clear plans to manage any crisis situation and to communicate effectively with their different stakeholders, to ensure consistent, regular, and transparent updates during a crisis. They should train their spokespersons and communication teams to handle media inquiries effectively. Establishing effective crisis communication protocols in post-COVID-19 period is crucial for maintaining transparency, managing public perception, and ensuring a coordinated response. By carefully planning and implementing these crisis communication protocols, organizations can respond effectively to challenges, maintain trust, and mitigate the impact of crises on both internal and external stakeholders. Managers need to regularly review and update these protocols to adapt to evolving circumstances and lessons learned from each crisis. In this section, we provide a brief guide to help managers develop robust crisis communication protocols to deal with any major crisis situation in future.

Cross-functional crisis team: Create a cross-functional crisis communication team with representatives from PR, legal, HR, and relevant departments with clearly defined roles and responsibilities for each team member.

Preparedness training through regular drills: Conduct regular crisis communication drills to test the effectiveness of the protocols. Provide training for team members on crisis communication best practices.

Risk assessment and scenario planning: Conduct a thorough risk assessment to identify potential crises. Develop response plans for various crisis scenarios, including public health emergencies.

Communication flow and channels: Establish a clear chain of command for communication during a crisis. Identify primary and secondary communication channels for both internal and external stakeholders.

Real-time media monitoring: Deploy advanced real-time media monitoring tools to stay informed about public sentiment and news coverage. Monitor social media for mentions and discussions related to the crisis.

Documentation and messaging: Prepare templates for press releases, internal communications, and other messaging in advance. Ensure consistency in messaging across all communication channels.

Spokesperson media training: Provide media training for designated spokespeople. Teach spokespeople to stay on-message and avoid speculation during crises to prevent possible public relations disasters and blow backs to the business.

Internal communication for employee notifications: Establish protocols for quickly notifying employees about the situation. Use multiple channels to disseminate information internally. Communicate openly and honestly with stakeholders. Acknowledge mistakes and communicate corrective actions, if applicable.

Legal and regulatory compliance: Engage professional legal counsel to ensure that communications comply with laws and regulations. Be aware of any reporting requirements imposed by relevant authorities.

Stakeholder engagement: Keep key stakeholders, such as partners and suppliers, informed and engaged. Develop a strategy for notifying customers about the crisis.

Designated communication center (physical and/or virtual): Establish a designated communication center for crisis management. Ensure that the communication center is available around the clock, especially during a crisis.

Provide regular updates: Provide regular updates to keep stakeholders informed of developments. Schedule media briefings to address questions and concerns.

Post-crisis review: Conduct a comprehensive review after the crisis to evaluate the effectiveness of the communication plan. Identify areas for improvement and incorporate lessons learned into future protocols.

Community outreach: Develop strategies for engaging with the local community if the crisis has community implications. Consider community support initiatives to demonstrate corporate social responsibility.

Remote communication protocols: Establish protocols for remote communication in case team members are not physically present. Ensure the security of virtual communication channels to prevent leaks or misinformation.

Dedicated crisis website: Create a dedicated crisis website or hub with essential information for stakeholders. Update the website in real-time with the latest information.

Coordination with government and health authorities: Coordinate closely with relevant government and health authorities. Collaborate on joint statements when appropriate.

Employee support programs: Offer employee assistance programs for mental health and well-being during and after the crisis. Provide channels for employees to share their concerns and receive available support if needed.

8.9 Test and revise crisis management plans

Organizations need to regularly test their crisis response plan through simulations and desktop exercises by conducting post-incident analyses after each crisis or simulation, to identify areas for improvement and make necessary revisions. Testing and revising crisis plans, especially in the context of post-COVID-19, is crucial to ensure they remain effective and relevant. In this section, we provide a step-by-step guide to test and revise crisis management plans. By following these steps, managers can systematically test and revise their crisis plans in post-COVID-19 period – ensuring that their organization is well-prepared for future challenges.

Review the current plans: Start by thoroughly reviewing the existing crisis management plan. Ensure that it reflects the lessons learned during the COVID-19 pandemic.

Assess the impact of COVID-19: Evaluate how COVID-19 specifically impacted the organization. Consider changes in operations, communication challenges, and any shortcomings in the response.

Gather comments and feedback: Collect feedback from key stakeholders, including employees, managers, and external partners. This can provide valuable insights into the strengths and weaknesses of the current plan.

Conduct risk assessment: Identify any new risks that may have emerged as a result of the pandemic. Consider changes in the business environment, supply chain disruptions, and the impact on workforce availability.

Update contact information: Ensure that contact information for key personnel, stakeholders, and emergency services is up-to-date. This includes phone numbers, email addresses, and other relevant communication channels.

Review communication protocols: Assess the effectiveness of communication channels during the pandemic. Consider implementing new tools or strategies to enhance communication during crises.

Scenario-based testing: Conduct scenario-based testing to simulate various crisis situations. This can help identify gaps in the plan and ensure that teams are familiar with their roles and responsibilities.

Incorporate remote work considerations: If remote work has become a more significant part of business operations, ensure that the crisis plan accommodates remote work challenges. Include provisions for virtual communication, coordination, and support.

Training and awareness: Provide ongoing training to employees to ensure they understand the revised crisis plan. This includes training on new technologies, communication tools, and updated response procedures.

Collaborate with external partners: If the organization works closely with external partners or vendors, collaborate with them to align crisis response strategies. Ensure that there is a clear understanding of each party's role in a crisis situation.

Seek professional assistance: Consider engaging with crisis management professionals or consultants who can provide an objective assessment of the plan and offer insights into best practices.

Legal and regulatory compliance: Review and update the crisis plan to ensure compliance with any new legal or regulatory requirements that may have emerged as a result of the pandemic. Establish a robust system for documenting incidents and the organization's response. This documentation is crucial for post-crisis analysis and continuous improvement.

Continuous improvement: Crisis management is an evolving process. Regularly revisit and update the crisis plan based on feedback, changes in the business environment, and emerging best practices. Schedule regular crisis drills and exercises to test the effectiveness of the plan. This helps identify areas that may need further refinement.

8.10 Collaborate more effectively with key stakeholders

Businesses should build and strengthen their existing relationships with local government agencies, industry associations, and peer businesses, to have access to their invaluable resources and insights during future crises. Collaborating with stakeholders effectively is crucial for the success of any organization, especially in the post-COVID-19 era. In this section, we discuss some strategies to enhance collaboration with key stakeholders, especially during and after a major crisis. By implementing these strategies, organizations can enhance their collaboration with stakeholders, fostering a more inclusive and productive working relationship in the post-pandemic era.

Clear communication: Establish clear and open lines of communication. Use various channels, such as video conferencing, collaboration tools, and regular updates, to keep stakeholders informed about the organization's activities and decisions.

Regular check-ins: Schedule regular check-ins with key stakeholders. These can be in the form of virtual meetings, webinars, or town hall sessions to discuss progress, challenges, and upcoming initiatives.

Utilize collaboration tools: Leverage collaboration tools and platforms that facilitate communication and document sharing. Platforms like Slack, Microsoft Teams, or Asana can enhance real-time collaboration and keep everyone on the same page.

Engage in two-way communication: Encourage feedback from stakeholders. Actively seek their input on key decisions, projects, and strategies. This not only shows that their opinions are valued but also provides valuable insights.

Foster a culture of transparency: Share relevant information about the organization's performance, challenges, and future plans. Transparency builds trust and confidence among stakeholders.

Customize communication: Recognize that different stakeholders may have different preferences for communication. Tailor the communication strategies to accommodate various needs, whether it's through email updates, newsletters, or direct meetings.

Establish clear expectations: Clearly define roles, responsibilities, and expectations for both the organization and stakeholders. This clarity helps avoid misunderstandings and ensures everyone is aligned toward common goals.

Virtual engagement opportunities: Organize virtual events, webinars, or workshops to engage with stakeholders. These events provide opportunities for interaction, idea sharing, and networking, fostering a sense of community.

Adapt to remote work realities: Acknowledge and adapt to the remote work environment that may persist in post-COVID-19 period. Utilize virtual collaboration tools and ensure that processes are in place to support effective remote collaboration.

Continuous improvement: Regularly evaluate and seek feedback on the collaborative processes. Use this information to make continuous improvements and refine collaboration strategies over time.

Inclusive decision-making: Involve stakeholders in decision-making processes, especially those that directly impact them. This inclusivity not only strengthens relationships but also leads to better-informed decisions.

Build personal connections: Take the time to build personal connections with key stakeholders. Understanding their perspectives, motivations, and concerns can strengthen the working relationship.

Provide support and resources: Offer support and resources to stakeholders as needed. This could include providing training, access to relevant information, or assistance in overcoming challenges.

Flexibility and adaptability: Be flexible and adaptable in the approach. Recognize that circumstances may change, and the organization needs to respond accordingly. Solicit feedback on how the organization can adapt to evolving situations.

Celebrate successes: Acknowledge and celebrate achievements, milestones, and successes. Recognizing and appreciating the contributions of stakeholders builds a positive and collaborative atmosphere.

8.11 Stay informed and monitor trends

Businesses should stay informed about emerging risks and trends that could impact their industry and own operations, by continuously monitoring global events, economic indicators, and market conditions, to make proactive adjustments to their strategy. Staying informed and monitoring trends is essential for businesses and individuals to adapt to the changing landscape. By employing these strategies, they can create a robust system for staying informed and monitoring trends in post-COVID-19 era, allowing the organizations and managers to make informed decisions and stay ahead of the curve. In this section, we describe some strategies to help businesses and managers stay informed to keep them prepared to handle any significant crisis or event.

Diversify information sources: Don't rely on a single source for information. Follow a diverse range of reputable news outlets, industry publications, blogs, and research reports to get a comprehensive view of trends.

Use aggregator tools: Consider using news aggregator tools and apps that compile news from various sources. Examples include Flipboard, Feedly, or news apps that allow you to customize your content.

Set up Google alerts: Create Google Alerts for specific keywords related to your industry or interests. This will allow you to receive email notifications when new content matching the chosen keywords is published online.

Follow influencers and thought leaders: Identify and follow influencers, thought leaders, and experts in the industry on social media platforms. They often share valuable insights and trends that can help everyone stay ahead.

Participate in webinars and virtual events: Attend webinars, virtual conferences, and industry events. These events often feature expert speakers discussing the latest trends and insights in various fields.

Join professional associations and networks: Become a member of professional associations and networks related to the industry. These organizations often provide newsletters, reports, and events that can keep the practitioners informed about industry trends.

Network with peers: Engage in discussions with peers and colleagues. Networking can provide firsthand insights into industry developments and emerging trends.

Monitor social media: Stay active on social media platforms where industry discussions take place. Platforms like LinkedIn and Twitter are particularly useful for professional networking and staying updated on industry news.

Read industry reports and research: Keep an eye on industry reports and research studies. Many organizations and research firms release reports on market trends, consumer behavior, and other relevant topics. Subscribe to newsletters from reputable sources in the industry to receive curated content directly in your inbox, saving time while staying informed.

Continuous learning: Invest time in continuous learning. Attend online courses, workshops, and training programs to enhance your knowledge and skills in the field.

Evaluate and adapt: Regularly assess the information received and be willing to adapt relevant strategies and plans based on emerging trends. Flexibility is key in a rapidly changing post-COVID-19 environment.

Follow government updates: Stay informed about government policies and regulations that may impact the industry. Government websites, press releases, and regulatory updates are valuable sources of information.

Stay informed about global events: Be aware of global events and their potential impact on the industry. Economic, political, and social changes around the world can have ripple effects on various sectors.

Utilize analytics tools: Use analytics tools to monitor online engagement and trends. Tools like Google Analytics, social media analytics, and trend analysis tools can provide valuable data on what topics are gaining traction.

8.12 Establish a business continuity management system (BCMS)

Businesses may find it useful to implement a BCMS based on ISO 22301 standards to ensure a structured and systematic approach to business continuity and crisis management. By taking these steps, businesses can proactively prepare themselves for future crises, enhancing their ability to respond effectively and safeguard their operations, employees, and stakeholders. Preparedness and resilience are essential attributes for long-term success in an ever-changing business landscape. Establishing a BCMS is crucial to ensure that organizations can continue their critical operations and services in the face of disruptions, such as those experienced during and post-COVID-19 period. By following these steps, managers can establish a comprehensive BCMS to help their organizations effectively respond to and recover from disruptions, such as those experienced in the post-COVID-19 era. Regularly reviewing and updating the BCMS would ensure its ongoing effectiveness and relevance. In this section, we provide a step-by-step guide to help managers establish a robust and effective BCMS in their organizations.

Secure leadership commitment and support: Ensure that top management understands the importance of business continuity and is actively involved in its implementation.

Establish a business continuity management (BCM) team: Form a dedicated BCM team responsible for developing, implementing, and maintaining the BCMS. This team should include representatives from key departments and functions.

Conduct a business impact analysis (BIA): Identify critical business processes and functions. Conduct a BIA to assess the potential impact of disruptions on these processes. This analysis helps prioritize recovery efforts.

Risk assessment: Perform a comprehensive risk assessment to identify potential threats and vulnerabilities. This includes natural disasters, cyber threats, supply chain disruptions, and other risks that could affect your organization.

Develop a business continuity policy: Draft a business continuity policy that outlines the organization's commitment to maintaining critical functions during disruptions. Ensure that this policy aligns with the overall business objectives.

Create a BCP: Develop a detailed BCP that includes strategies and procedures for responding to identified risks and disruptions. This plan should address both short-term response and long-term recovery.

Incident response plan: Develop an incident response plan to guide the organization's immediate actions in the event of a disruption. This plan should include communication protocols, emergency response procedures, and initial recovery steps.

Crisis communication plan: Establish a crisis communication plan to ensure timely and effective communication with internal and external stakeholders during a crisis. Clearly define roles and responsibilities for communication.

Training and awareness: Train employees at all levels on their roles and responsibilities in the event of a disruption. Conduct regular drills and exercises to test the effectiveness of the BCM system and improve staff readiness.

Testing and exercising: Regularly test and conduct exercises to evaluate the effectiveness of the BCM system. This includes tabletop exercises, simulated drills, and full-scale tests to identify areas for improvement.

Document and update: Document all aspects of the BCM system, including plans, procedures, and lessons learned from exercises. Regularly review and update the documentation to ensure it remains current and relevant.

Supplier and partner engagement: Engage with key suppliers and partners to ensure they have their own BCPs. Collaborate on strategies to address shared risks and dependencies.

Technology and data protection: Address technology resilience and data protection in the BCM system. Ensure that IT systems are capable of supporting critical functions and that data is securely backed up and recoverable.

Regulatory compliance: Ensure that the BCM system complies with relevant regulatory requirements and industry standards. Stay informed about any changes in regulations that may impact the BCP.

Continuous improvement: Establish a process for continuous improvement. Regularly review and update the BCM system based on changes in the business environment, emerging risks, and lessons learned from incidents.

8.13 Conclusion

COVID-19 has proven to be a dynamic and evolving crisis, marked by subsequent waves of infections and the emergence of new strains. Navigating this landscape requires ongoing vigilance, research, and adaptation of strategies. Effective vaccination campaigns, vigilant surveillance, and international cooperation will continue to be essential tools in managing the evolving COVID-19 until widespread immunity is achieved and the threat of new strains is minimized. Preparing for unexpected crises like the COVID-19 pandemic requires a comprehensive and adaptable strategy. For example, businesses need to regularly conduct risk assessments to identify potential threats and develop scenarios that simulate various crisis situations, allowing for better preparedness. They also need to create robust BCPs that outline procedures for maintaining essential operations during a crisis, which should be tested regularly and updated based on lessons learned and changes in the business environment. Businesses should also maintain a strong financial position with sufficient reserves to cover operational expenses during challenging times. They should try to diversify revenue streams to reduce dependence on specific markets or products.

Businesses should also try to diversify their suppliers and build strong relationships with alternative sources to avoid supply chain disruptions. They should also develop contingency plans for supply chain disruptions and regularly review and update them. The pandemic has highlighted the importance of investing in robust digital infrastructure to enable remote work and maintain operations during disruptions. Hence, more businesses should embrace digital tools for collaboration, communication, and customer engagement. Another lesson from the pandemic has been about the importance of managing employee well-being to ensure motivation and productivity during challenging times. Hence, businesses should prioritize employee health and safety and provide mental health support by establishing flexible work arrangements and remote work policies. They may also provide cross-functional training to their employees to ensure multiple team members can perform critical functions. Moreover, establishing redundancy in key roles and systems may also help mitigate the impact of personnel shortages or system failures during challenging times. Similarly, providing scenario-based training exercises would help prepare employees for various crisis situations.

Businesses should also develop a clear and transparent communication strategy and plans for both internal and external stakeholders, to provide regular updates during crises to maintain trust and manage expectations. Similarly, it is very important for managers to keep informed about relevant regulations and compliance requirements to ensure that the business is adaptable to changes in regulatory environments while remaining compliant with the regulatory and legal requirements. They should also evaluate the effectiveness of various response mechanisms and adjust their strategies accordingly. The pandemic also highlighted the importance of collaborations and relationships with external partners, hence businesses should foster relationships with other businesses, industry associations, and government agencies. This would help them collaborate with others on information sharing, resource allocation, and joint crisis response efforts, to improve the quality of collective response to any challenges.

Businesses should also integrate their sustainability practices and social responsibility into the core of the business, which would help them demonstrate a commitment to broader societal goals, which can enhance resilience and reputation. Finally, they should regularly review and update their crisis management plans based on evolving risks and lessons learned, by developing a culture of continuous improvement and adaptation. By proactively addressing these aspects, businesses can enhance their ability to navigate unexpected crises and emerge more resilient on the other side. Flexibility, adaptability, and a forward-looking mindset are key components of effective crisis preparedness for businesses in the post-pandemic era.

References

Adedoyin, O. B., & Soykan, E. (2023). COVID-19 pandemic and online learning: The challenges and opportunities. *Interactive Learning Environments, 31*(2), 863–875.

Ades, A. S. (2020). The effective of health communication about the awareness of COVID-19 through social media. *Social Medicine, 13*(3), 118–126.

Adongo, P. B., Tabong, P. T. N., Asampong, E., Ansong, J., Robalo, M., & Adanu, R. M. (2016). Preparing towards preventing and containing an Ebola virus disease outbreak: What socio-cultural practices may affect containment efforts in Ghana? *PLoS Neglected Tropical Diseases, 10*(7), e0004852. https://doi.org/10.1371/journal.pntd.0004852

Agarwal, P., Swami, S., & Malhotra, S. K. (2022). Artificial intelligence adoption in the post COVID-19 new-normal and role of smart technologies in transforming business: A review. *Journal of Science and Technology Policy Management.* https://doi.org/10.1108/JSTPM-08-2021-0122

Aguinis, H., Villamor, I., & Gabriel, K. P. (2020). Understanding employee responses to COVID-19: A behavioral corporate social responsibility perspective. *Management Research: Journal of the Iberoamerican Academy of Management, 18*(4), 421–438.

Agusto, F. B., Teboh-Ewungkem, M. I., & Gumel, A. B. (2015). Mathematical assessment of the effect of traditional beliefs and customs on the transmission dynamics of the 2014 ebola outbreaks. *BMC Medicine, 13*(1), 1–17. https://doi.org/10.1186/s12916-015-0318-3

Ahmed, F., Zhao, F., & Faraz, N. A. (2020). How and when does inclusive leadership curb psychological distress during a crisis? Evidence from the COVID-19 outbreak. *Frontiers in Psychology, 11*, 1898.

Aknin, L. B., Andretti, B., Goldszmidt, R., Helliwell, J. F., Petherick, A., De Neve, J. E., Dunn, E. W., Fancourt, D., Goldberg, E., Jones, S. P., Karadag, O., Karam, E., Layard, R., Saxena, S., Thornton, E., Whillans, A., & Zaki, J. (2022). Policy stringency and mental health during the COVID-19 pandemic: A longitudinal analysis of data from 15 countries. *The Lancet Public Health, 7*(5), e417–e426.

Alcedo, J., Cavallo, A., Dwyer, B., Mishra, P., & Spilimbergo, A. (2022). *E-commerce during COVID: Stylized facts from 47 economies* (No. w29729). National Bureau of Economic Research.

Al-Hunaiyyan, A., Alhajri, R., & Bimba, A. (2021). Towards an efficient integrated distance and blended learning model: How to minimise the impact of COVID-19 on education. *International Journal of Interactive Mobile Technologies, 15*(10), 173–193.

Allel, K., Tapia-Muñoz, T., & Morris, W. (2020). Country-level factors associated with the early spread of COVID-19 cases at 5, 10 and 15 days since the onset. *Global Public Health, 15*(11), 1589–1602.

Allen, J., Mahamed, F., & Williams, K. (2022). Disparities in education: E-learning and COVID-19, who matters? *Child & Youth Services, 41*(3), 208–210.

Alwashmi, M. F. (2020). The use of digital health in the detection and management of COVID-19. *International Journal of Environmental Research and Public Health, 17*(8), 2906.

Amer, F., Hammoud, S., Farran, B., Boncz, I., & Endrei, D. (2021). Assessment of countries' preparedness and lockdown effectiveness in fighting COVID-19. *Disaster Medicine and Public Health Preparedness, 15*(2), e15–e22.

Amer, S. A., Shah, J., Abd-Ellatif, E. E., & El Maghawry, H. A. (2022). COVID-19 vaccine uptake among physicians during the second wave of COVID-19 pandemic: Attitude, intentions, and determinants: A cross-sectional study. *Frontiers in Public Health, 10*, 823217.

Amir, H. (2022). Strategies in preventing the transmission of COVID-19 a quarantine, isolation, lockdown, tracing, testing and treatment (3t): Literature review. *Asia Pacific Journal of Health Management, 17*(2), 1–6.

Ancarani, A., Ayach, A., Di Mauro, C., Gitto, S., & Mancuso, P. (2016). Does religious diversity in health team composition affect efficiency? Evidence from Dubai. *British Journal of Management, 27*(4), 740–759.

Andrulli, R., & Gerards, R. (2023). How new ways of working during COVID-19 affect employee well-being via technostress, need for recovery, and work engagement. *Computers in Human Behavior, 139*, 107560.

Aronna, M. S., Guglielmi, R., & Moschen, L. M. (2021). A model for COVID-19 with isolation, quarantine and testing as control measures. *Epidemics, 34*, 100437.

Ashcroft, P., Lehtinen, S., & Bonhoeffer, S. (2022). Test-trace-isolate-quarantine (TTIQ) intervention strategies after symptomatic COVID-19 case identification. *PLoS ONE, 17*(2), e0263597.

Ashraf, B. N. (2020). Economic impact of government interventions during the COVID-19 pandemic: International evidence from financial markets. *Journal of Behavioral and Experimental Finance, 27*, 100371.

Augustin, P., Sokolovski, V., Subrahmanyam, M. G., & Tomio, D. (2022). In sickness and in debt: The COVID-19 impact on sovereign credit risk. *Journal of Financial Economics, 143*(3), 1251–1274.

Australian Treasury. (2023). Independent Evaluation of the JobKeeper Payment: Consultation Paper (16 June 2023). https://treasury.gov.au/sites/default/files/2023-06/c2023-407908.pdf

Backhaus, I., Sisenop, F., Begotaraj, E., Cachia, J., Capolongo, S., Carta, M. G., Jakubauskiene, M., Jevtic, M., Nakov, V., Pirlog, M. C., Grbic, D. S., Vinko, M., Kusturica, M. P., Morganti, A., & Lindert, J. (2021). Resilience and coping with COVID-19: The COPERS study. *International Journal of Public Health, 66*, 1604007.

Balser, J., Ryu, J., Hood, M., Kaplan, G., Perlin, J., & Siegel, B. (2021). Care systems COVID-19 impact assessment: Lessons learned and compelling needs. *NAM Perspectives.* Discussion Paper, National Academy of Medicine, Washington, DC. https://doi.org/10.31478/202104d

Bates, C. R., Nicholson, L. M., Rea, E. M., Hagy, H. A., & Bohnert, A. M. (2021). Life interrupted: Family routines buffer stress during the COVID-19 pandemic. *Journal of Child and Family Studies, 30*(11), 2641–2651.

Bayram, A. B., & Shields, T. (2021). Who trusts the WHO? Heuristics and Americans' trust in the world health organization during the COVID-19 pandemic. *Social Science Quarterly*, *102*(5), 2312–2330.

Belletsky, M. R., Anstett, C., & Teitelbaum, M. A. (2020). Life and financial planning in the time of COVID-19. *Journal of Financial Service Professionals*, *74*(4), 41–53.

Beninger, S., & Francis, J. N. (2022). Resources for business resilience in a COVID-19 world: A community-centric approach. *Business Horizons*, *65*(2), 227–238.

Bernardo, T., Sobkowich, K. E., Forrest, R. O., Stewart, L. S., D'Agostino, M., Perez Gutierrez, E., & Gillis, D. (2021). Collaborating in the time of COVID-19: The scope and scale of innovative responses to a global pandemic. *JMIR Public Health and Surveillance*, *7*(2), e25935. https://doi.org/10.2196/25935.

Bhatt, V., Chakraborty, S., Chakravorty, T., & Studies, E. (2020). Importance of digitech adoption for providing efficient healthcare services during COVID-19. *International Journal on Emerging Technologies*, *11*(3), 1–13.

Bisco, J. M., Fier, S. G., & Pooser, D. M. (2020). Business interruption insurance and COVID-19: Coverage and issues and public policy implications. *Journal of Insurance Regulation*, *39*(5), 1–24.

Blumenfeld, S., Anderson, G., & Hooper, V. (2020). Covid-19 and employee surveillance. *New Zealand Journal of Employment Relations*, *45*(2), 42–56.

Bolislis, W. R., De Lucia, M. L., Dolz, F., Mo, R., Nagaoka, M., Rodriguez, H., Woon, M. L., Yu, W., & Kühler, T. C. (2021). Regulatory agilities in the time of covid-19: Overview, trends, and opportunities. *Clinical Therapeutics*, *43*(1), 124–139.

Borisova, L. V., Martinussen, P. E., Rydland, H. T., Stornes, P., & Eikemo, T. A. (2017). Public evaluation of health services across 21 European countries: The role of culture. *Scandinavian Journal of Public Health*, *45*(2), 132–139.

Brueck, H. (2020). Sweden's gamble on coronavirus herd immunity couldn't work in the US – and it may not work in Sweden. *Business Insider*. 2 May 2020. https://www.businessinsider.com/sweden-coronavirus-strategy-explained-culture-of-trust-and-obedience-2020-4.

Bryant, J., Child, F., Dorn, E., Espinosa, J., Hall, S., Kola-Oyeneyin, T., Lim, C., Panier, F., Sarakatsannis, J., Schmautzer, D., Ungur, S., & Woord, B. (2022). How COVID-19 caused a global learning crisis? *McKinsey & Company*, 1–22. https://www.mckinsey.com/industries/education/our-insights/how-covid-19-caused-a-global-learning-crisis.

Bryant, T. J., Vertinsky, H., & Smart, C. (2007). Globalization and international communicable crises: A case study of SARS. In D. E. Gibbons (Ed.), *Communicable crises: Prevention, response, and recovery in the global arena* (pp. 265–300). Information Age Publishing.

Bukovska, G., Mezgaile, A., & Klepers, A. (2021). The pressure of technological innovations in meeting and event industry under the COVID-19 influence. *Environment, Technologies. Resources. Proceedings of the International Scientific and Practical Conference*, *2*, 44–50.

Bullock, A., Colvin, A. D., & Jackson, M. S. (2022). Zoom fatigue in the age of COVID-19. *Journal of Social Work in the Global Community*, *7*(1), 1–9. https://doi.org/10.5590/JSWGC.2022.07.1.01.

Burki, T. K. (2020). COVID-19: Consequences for higher education. *The Lancet Oncology*, *21*(6), 758. https://doi.org/10.1016/S1470-2045(20)30287-4.

Cadeddu, C., Rosano, A., Villani, L., Coiante, G. B., Minicucci, I., Pascucci, D., & De Waure, C. (2022). Planning and organization of the COVID-19 vaccination campaign: An overview of eight European countries. *Vaccines*, *10*(10), 1631.

Callaway, E. (2023). The next generation of coronavirus vaccines. *Nature, 614,* 22–25.

Çelik, E., Biçener, E., & Makas, S. (2023). Relationship between anxiety sensitivity, death anxiety, and resilience in the age of pandemics and lifelong learning. *International Journal of Educational Research Review, 8*(2), 289–302.

Chae, D., Kim, J., Kim, K., Ryu, J., Asami, K., & Doorenbos, A. Z. (2023). An immersive virtual reality simulation for cross-cultural communication skills: Development and feasibility. *Clinical Simulation in Nursing, 77,* 13–22.

Chang, S. E., Brown, C., Handmer, J., Helgeson, J., Kajitani, Y., Keating, A., Noy, I., Watson, M., Derakhshan, S., Kim, J., & Roa-Henriquez, A. (2022). Business recovery from disasters: Lessons from natural hazards and the COVID-19 pandemic. *International Journal of Disaster Risk Reduction, 80,* 103191.

Chang, C. L., McAleer, M., & Wong, W. K. (2020). Risk and financial management of COVID-19 in business, economics and finance. *Journal of Risk and Financial Management, 13*(5), 102.

Charitos, I. A., Ballini, A., Lovero, R., Castellaneta, F., Colella, M., Scacco, S., Cantore, S., Arrigoni, R., Mastrangelo, F., & Dioguardi, M. (2022). Update on COVID-19 and effectiveness of a vaccination campaign in a global context. *International Journal of Environmental Research and Public Health, 19*(17), 10712.

Chaturvedi, K., Vishwakarma, D. K., & Singh, N. (2021). COVID-19 and its impact on education, social life and mental health of students: A survey. *Children and Youth Services Review, 121,* 105866.

Chau, C. H., Strope, J. D., & Figg, W. D. (2020). COVID-19 clinical diagnostics and testing technology. *Pharmacotherapy: The Journal of Human Pharmacology and Drug Therapy, 40*(8), 857–868.

Cheema-Fox, A., LaPerla, B. R., Wang, H., & Serafeim, G. (2021). Corporate resilience and response to COVID-19. *Journal of Applied Corporate Finance, 33*(2), 24–40.

Cheng, S., Zhao, Y., Kaminga, A. C., Wang, X., Zhang, X., & Xu, H. (2022). COVID-19 containment: Comparisons and suggestions for global response. *Inquiry: The Journal of Health Care Organization, Provision, and Financing, 59,* 00469580221086142.

Chernoff, A., & Warman, C. (2023). COVID-19 and implications for automation. *Applied Economics, 55*(17), 1939–1957.

Chesbrough, H. (2020). To recover faster from covid-19, open up: Managerial implications from an open innovation perspective. *Industrial Marketing Management, 88,* 410–413.

Chinazzi, M., Davis, J. T., Ajelli, M., Gioannini, C., Litvinova, M., Merler, S., Pastore y Piontti, A., Mu, K., Rossi, L., Sun, K., Viboud, C., Xiong, X., Yu, H., Halloran, M. E., Longini, I. M., & Vespignani, A. (2020). The effect of travel restrictions on the spread of the 2019 novel coronavirus (COVID-19) outbreak. *Science, 368*(6489), 395–400.

Chu, I. Y. H., Alam, P., Larson, H. J., & Lin, L. (2020). Social consequences of mass quarantine during epidemics: A systematic review with implications for the COVID-19 response. *Journal of Travel Medicine, 27*(7), taaa192.

Chun, H. K., Comyn, P., & Moreno da Fonseca, P. (2021). Skills development in the time of COVID-19: Taking stock of the initial responses in technical and vocational education and training. International Labour Office. http://hdl.voced.edu.au/10707/565426.

Chung, S. C., Marlow, S., Tobias, N., Alogna, A., Alogna, I., You, S. L., Khunti, K., McKee, M., Michie, S., & Pillay, D. (2021). Lessons from countries implementing find, test, trace, isolation and support policies in the rapid response of the COVID-19 pandemic: A systematic review. *BMJ Open, 11*(7), e047832.

Church, A. T. (2000). Culture and personality: Toward an integrated cultural trait psychology. *Journal of Personality, 68*(4), 651–703.

Cirera, X., Cruz, M., Davies, E., Grover, A., Iacovone, L., Cordova, J. E. L., Medvedev, D., Maduko, F. O., Nayyar, G., Reyes Ortega, S., & Torres, J. (2021). Policies to support businesses through the COVID-19 shock: A firm level perspective. *The World Bank Research Observer, 36*(1), 41–66.

Clay, S. L., Woodson, M. J., Mazurek, K., & Antonio, B. (2021). Racial disparities and COVID-19: Exploring the relationship between race/ethnicity, personal factors, health access/affordability, and conditions associated with an increased severity of COVID-19. *Race and Social Problems, 13*, 279–291.

Coelho, C. M., Suttiwan, P., Arato, N., & Zsido, A. N. (2020). On the nature of fear and anxiety triggered by COVID-19. *Frontiers in Psychology, 11*, 581314.

Colleoni, E., Romenti, S., Valentini, C., Badham, M., Choi, S. I., Kim, S., & Jin, Y. (2022). Does culture matter? Measuring cross-country perceptions of CSR communication campaigns about COVID-19. *Sustainability, 14*(2), 889.

Cortes, G. M., & Forsythe, E. (2023). Heterogeneous labor market impacts of the COVID-19 pandemic. *ILR Review, 76*(1), 30–55.

Cox, P. L., Friedman, B. A., & Tribunella, T. (2011). Relationships among cultural dimensions, national gross domestic product, and environmental sustainability. *Journal of Applied Business and Economics, 12*(6), 46–56.

Crawford, J., Butler-Henderson, K., Rudolph, J., Glowatz, M., Burton, R., Magni, P. A., & Lam, S. (2020). COVID-19: 20 countries' higher education intra-period digital pedagogy responses. *Journal of Applied Learning & Teaching, 3*(1), 1–20.

Cunha, M. P. E., Simpson, A. V., Clegg, S. R., & Rego, A. (2019). Speak! Paradoxical effects of a managerial culture of speaking up. *British Journal of Management, 30*(4), 829–846.

Curtis, V., Dreibelbis, R., Sidibe, M., Cardosi, J., Sara, J., Bonell, C., Mwambuli, K., Moulik, S. G., White, S., & Aunger, R. (2020). How to set up government-led national hygiene communication campaigns to combat COVID-19: A strategic blueprint. *BMJ Global Health, 5*(8), e002780.

Dahlke, J., Bogner, K., Becker, M., Schlaile, M. P., Pyka, A., & Ebersberger, B. (2021). Crisis-driven innovation and fundamental human needs: A typological framework of rapid-response COVID-19 innovations. *Technological Forecasting and Social Change, 169*, 120799.

Daneshfar, Z., Asokan-Ajitha, A., Sharma, P., & Malik, A. (2023). Work-from-home (WFH) during COVID-19 pandemic–A netnographic investigation using Twitter data. *Information Technology & People, 36*(5), 2161–2186.

Daniels, R. A., Miller, L. A., Mian, M. Z., & Black, S. (2022). One size does NOT fit all: Understanding differences in perceived organizational support during the COVID-19 pandemic. *Business and Society Review, 127*, 193–222.

Danisman, G. O., Demir, E., & Zaremba, A. (2021). Financial resilience to the COVID-19 pandemic: The role of banking market structure. *Applied Economics, 53*(39), 4481–4504.

De Soyres, F., Santacreu, A. M., & Young, H. (2022). Fiscal policy and excess inflation during Covid-19: A cross-country view. *FEDS Notes. Washington: Board of Governors of the Federal Reserve System* (15 July 2022). https://doi.org/10.17016/2380-7172.3083.

De Vries, P. (2020). COVID-19 versus Japan's culture of collectivism. *The Japan Times*, 22 May 2020. https://www.japantimes.co.jp/opinion/2020/05/22/commentary/japan-commentary/covid-19-versus-japans-culture-collectivism/

De Witte, M. (2020). How a yellow fever outbreak reshaped New Orleans. *Futurity*, 26 March 2020. https://www.futurity.org/yellow-fever-pandemics-anxiety-2317582-2/

Dejardin, M., Raposo, M. L., Ferreira, J. J., Fernandes, C. I., Veiga, P. M., & Farinha, L. (2023). The impact of dynamic capabilities on SME performance during COVID-19. *Review of Managerial Science*, 17, 1703–1729.

Delardas, O., Kechagias, K. S., Pontikos, P. N., & Giannos, P. (2022). Socio-economic impacts and challenges of the coronavirus pandemic (COVID-19): An updated review. *Sustainability*, 14(15), 9699.

Devi, S. (2020). Travel restrictions hampering COVID-19 response. *The Lancet*, 395(10233), 1331–1332.

Dhama, K., Sharun, K., Tiwari, R., Dhawan, M., Emran, T. B., Rabaan, A. A., & Al-humaid, S. (2021). COVID-19 vaccine hesitancy–reasons and solutions to achieve a successful global vaccination campaign to tackle the ongoing pandemic. *Human Vaccines & Immunotherapeutics*, 17(10), 3495–3499.

Dietrich, A. M., Kuester, K., Müller, G. J., & Schoenle, R. (2022). News and uncertainty about COVID-19: Survey evidence and short-run economic impact. *Journal of Monetary Economics*, 129, S35–S51.

Dingel, J. I., & Neiman, B. (2020). How many jobs can be done at home? *Journal of Public Economic*, 189, 104235.

Donthu, N., & Gustafsson, A. (2020). Effects of COVID-19 on business and research. *Journal of Business Research*, 117, 284–289.

Dorn, E., Hancock, B., Sarakatsannis, J., & Viruleg, E. (2021). COVID-19 and education: The lingering effects of unfinished learning. *McKinsey & Company*, 1–15. https://www.mckinsey.com/industries/education/our-insights/covid-19-and-education-the-lingering-effects-of-unfinished-learning

Drane, C., Vernon, L., & O'Shea, S. (2020). The impact of 'learning at home' on the educational outcomes of vulnerable children in Australia during the COVID-19 pandemic. Literature review prepared by national centre for student equity in higher education. Curtin University.

Egede, L. E., Ruggiero, K. J., & Frueh, B. C. (2020). Ensuring mental health access for vulnerable populations in COVID era. *Journal of Psychiatric Research*, 129, 147.

Eikhof, D. R. (2020). COVID-19, inclusion and workforce diversity in the cultural economy: What now, what next? *Cultural Trends*, 29(3), 234–250.

Elali, W. (2021). The importance of strategic agility to business survival during corona crisis and beyond. *International Journal of Business Ethics and Governance*, 4(2), 1–8.

El-Shabasy, R. M., Nayel, M. A., Taher, M. M., Abdelmonem, R., Shoueir, K. R., & Kenawy, E. R. (2022). Three waves changes, new variant strains, and vaccination effect against COVID-19 pandemic. *International Journal of Biological Macromolecules*, 204, 161–168.

Espitia, A., Rocha, N., & Ruta, M. (2020). Covid-19 and food protectionism: The impact of The pandemic and export restrictions on world food markets. *World Bank Policy Research Working Paper* (9253).

Estanyol, E. (2022). Traditional festivals and COVID-19: Event management and digitalization in times of physical distancing. *Event Management*, 26(3), 647–659.

Falkner, R., Fasolo, B., Taj, U., Cnop-Nielson, A., Soane, E., & Chambers, S. (2022). How to upskill for 2022. *LSE Business Review* (31 January 2022). https://eprints.lse.ac.uk/114102/1/businessreview_2022_01_31_how_to_upskill_for.pdf

Farmaki, A., Hadjielias, E., Olya, H., Taheri, B., & Hadjielia Drotarova, M. (2022). CSR communication and international marketing: Insights from the COVID-19 pandemic. *International Marketing Review*. https://doi.org/10.1108/IMR-12-2021-0375.

Filetti, S. (2020). The COVID-19 pandemic requires a unified global response. *Endocrine*, *68*(1), 1–1.

Fong, K. H., & Snape, E. (2015). Empowering leadership, psychological empowerment and employee outcomes: Testing a multi-level mediating model. *British Journal of Management*, *26*(1), 126–138.

Forman, R., Atun, R., McKee, M., & Mossialos, E. (2020). 12 lessons learned from the management of the coronavirus pandemic. *Health Policy*, *124*(6), 577–580.

Fortier, N. (2020). COVID-19, gender inequality, and the responsibility of the state. *International Journal of Wellbeing*, *10*(3), 77–93.

Fox, J., & Bartholomae, S. (2020). Household finances, financial planning, and COVID-19. *Financial Planning Review*, *3*(4), e1103.

Fransen, J., Peralta, D. O., Vanelli, F., Edelenbos, J., & Olvera, B. C. (2022). The emergence of urban community resilience initiatives during the COVID-19 pandemic: An international exploratory study. *The European Journal of Development Research*, *34*, 432–454.

Fry, C. V., Cai, X., Zhang, Y., & Wagner, C. S. (2020). Consolidation in a crisis: Patterns of international collaboration in early COVID-19 research. *PLoS ONE*, *15*(7), e0236307.

Fu, Y., Jin, H., Xiang, H., & Wang, N. (2022). Optimal lockdown policy for vaccination during COVID-19 pandemic. *Finance Research Letters*, *45*, 102123.

Gamlath, S. (2017). Human development and national culture: A multivariate exploration. *Social Indicators Research*, *133*, 907–930.

García-Morales, V. J., Garrido-Moreno, A., & Martín-Rojas, R. (2021). The transformation of higher education after the COVID disruption: Emerging challenges in an online learning scenario. *Frontiers in Psychology*, *12*, 616059.

Gausman, J., & Langer, A. (2020). Sex and gender disparities in the COVID-19 pandemic. *Journal of Women's Health*, *29*(4), 465–466.

Gazi, T., & Gazis, A. (2020). Humanitarian aid in the age of COVID-19: A review of big data crisis analytics and the general data protection regulation. *International Review of the Red Cross*, *102*(913), 75–94.

Gibson, B., Schneider, J., Talamonti, D., & Forshaw, M. (2021). The impact of inequality on mental health outcomes during the COVID-19 pandemic: A systematic review. *Canadian Psychology/Psychologie Canadienne*, *62*(1), 101–126.

Girardi, P., Greco, L., & Ventura, L. (2022). Misspecified modeling of subsequent waves during COVID-19 outbreak: A change-point growth model. *Biometrical Journal*, *64*(3), 523–538.

Gottlieb, M., & Dyer, S. (2020). Information and disinformation: Social media in the COVID-19 crisis. *Academic Emergency Medicine*, *27*(7), 640–641.

Graham, M., Lambert, K. A., Weale, V., Stuckey, R., & Oakman, J. (2023). Working from home during the COVID 19 pandemic: A longitudinal examination of employees' sense of community and social support and impacts on self-rated health. *BMC Public Health*, *23*(1), 11.

Grimaud, J., & Legagneur, F. (2011). Community beliefs and fears during a cholera outbreak in Haiti. *Intervention: International Journal of Mental Health, Psychosocial Work & Counselling in Areas of Armed Conflict, 9*(1), 26–34.

Grimes, D. R. (2021). Medical disinformation and the unviable nature of COVID-19 conspiracy theories. *PLoS ONE, 16*(3), e0245900.

Gualano, M. R., Santoro, P. E., Borrelli, I., Rossi, M. F., Amantea, C., Tumminello, A., Daniele, A., Beccia, F., & Moscato, U. (2022). Employee participation in workplace vaccination campaigns: A systematic review and meta-analysis. *Vaccines, 10*(11), 1898.

Gundersen, C., Hake, M., Dewey, A., & Engelhard, E. (2021). Food insecurity during COVID-19. *Applied Economic Perspectives and Policy, 43*(1), 153–161.

Haelermans, C., Korthals, R., Jacobs, M., de Leeuw, S., Vermeulen, S., van Vugt, L., Aarts, B., Prokic-Breuer, T., van der Velden, R., van Wetten, S., & de Wolf, I. (2022). Sharp increase in inequality in education in times of the COVID-19-pandemic. *PLoS ONE, 17*(2), e0261114.

Hair, J. F., Risher, J. J., Sarstedt, M., & Ringle, C. M. (2019). When to use and how to report the results of PLS-SEM. *European Business Review, 31*(1), 2–24.

Hai, T. N., Van, Q. N., & Thi Tuyet, M. N. (2021). Digital transformation: Opportunities and challenges for leaders in the emerging countries in response to COVID-19 pandemic. *Emerging Science Journal, 5*(Special Issue), 21–36.

Hamilton, J. (2020). The strategic change matrix and business sustainability across COVID-19. *Sustainability, 12*(15), 6026.

Hamouche, S. (2020). COVID-19 and employees' mental health: Stressors, moderators and agenda for organizational actions. *Emerald Open Research, 2*, 15.

Hartley, D. M., & Perencevich, E. N. (2020). Public health interventions for COVID-19: Emerging evidence and implications for an evolving public health crisis. *JAMA, 323*(19), 1908–1909.

Hassoun, N. (2021). Against vaccine nationalism. *Journal of Medical Ethics, 47*(11), 773–774.

Headspace. (2020). Coping with COVID: The mental health impact on young people accessing headspace services (August 2020).

He, D., Ali, S. T., Fan, G., Gao, D., Song, H., Lou, Y., Zhao, S., Cowling, B. J., & Stone, L. (2022). Evaluation of effectiveness of global COVID-19 vaccination campaign. *Emerging Infectious Diseases, 28*(9), 1873–1876.

Hebbani, A. V., Pulakuntla, S., Pannuru, P., Aramgam, S., Badri, K. R., & Reddy, V. D. (2022). COVID-19: Comprehensive review on mutations and current vaccines. *Archives of Microbiology, 204*, 8.

Hite, L. M., & McDonald, K. S. (2020). Careers after COVID-19: Challenges and changes. *Human Resource Development International, 23*(4), 427–437.

Hobin, E., & Smith, B. (2020). Is another public health crisis brewing beneath the COVID-19 pandemic? *Canadian Journal of Public Health, 111*, 392–396.

Hoekman, B., Fiorini, M., & Yildirim, A. (2020). Export restrictions: A negative-sum policy response to the COVID-19 crisis. *Robert Schuman Centre for Advanced Studies Research Paper No. RSCAS, 23.*

Hofstede, G. (1980). *Culture's consequences: International differences in work-related values.* Sage Publications.

Hofstede, G. (1991). *Cultures and organizations: Software of the mind.* McGraw-Hill.

Hofstede, G. (2001). *Culture's consequences: Comparing values, behaviours, institutions and organizations across nations,* 2nd ed. Sage.

Hofstede, G., & Hofstede, G. J. (2005). *Cultures and organizations: Software of the mind*, 2nd ed. McGraw-Hill.

Hofstede, G., Hofstede, G. J., & Minkov, M. (2010). *Cultures and organizations: Software of the mind*, 3rd ed. McGraw-Hill.

Hwang, H., & Höllerer, M. A. (2020). The COVID-19 crisis and its consequences: Ruptures and transformations in the global institutional fabric. *The Journal of Applied Behavioral Science, 56*(3), 294–300.

Hwang, T. J., Rabheru, K., Peisah, C., Reichman, W., & Ikeda, M. (2020). Loneliness and social isolation during the COVID-19 pandemic. *International Psychogeriatrics, 32*(10), 1217–1220.

Ino, E., & Watanabe, K. (2022). Diversification of business risks due to social changes with COVID-19. *Journal of Disaster Research, 17*(1), 152–158.

Islam, A., Wahab, S. A., & Abdul Latiff, A. S. (2023). Can small and medium businesses endure the COVID-19 crisis through strategic philanthropy? *Management Matters, 20*(1), 16–35.

Jaafar, N. S., & Khan, N. (2022). Impact of digital marketing innovation in competitive event industry during COVID-19: Evidence from Malaysia and the United States. *International Journal of Interactive Mobile Technologies, 16*(9), 130–145.

Jacobs, J. L., Haidar, G., & Mellors, J. W. (2023). COVID-19: Challenges of viral variants. *Annual Review of Medicine, 74*, 31–53.

Jain, S. S., & Jain, S. P. (2018). Power distance belief and preference for transparency. *Journal of Business Research, 89*, 135–142.

Jain, A., Sarupria, A., & Kothari, A. (2020). The impact of COVID-19 on e-wallet's payments in Indian economy. *International Journal of Creative Research Thoughts, 8*(6), 2447–2454.

Jana, M., & Roy, T. (2021). The shifting geopolitics of coronavirus and the demise of neoliberalism with the big challenge for United nations. *Asia-Pacific Journal of Management Research and Innovation, 17*(1–2), 85–94.

Jia, Q., Guo, Y., Wang, G., & Barnes, S. J. (2020). Big data analytics in the fight against major public health incidents (including COVID-19): A conceptual framework. *International Journal of Environmental Research and Public Health, 17*(17), 6161.

Jones, B. L., Carter, M. C., Davis, C. M., & Wang, J. (2023). Diversity, equity, and inclusion: A decade of progress? *The Journal of Allergy and Clinical Immunology: In Practice, 11*(1), 116–125.

Kalimeris, P., Bithas, K., Richardson, C., & Nijkamp, P. (2020). Hidden linkages between resources and economy: A "Beyond-GDP" approach using alternative welfare indicators. *Ecological Economics, 169*, 106508.

Karalis, T. (2020). Planning and evaluation during educational disruption: Lessons learned from COVID-19 pandemic for treatment of emergencies in education. *European Journal of Education Studies, 7*(4), 125–142.

Karpen, I. O., & Conduit, J. (2020). Engaging in times of COVID-19 and beyond: Theorizing customer engagement through different paradigmatic lenses. *Journal of Service Management, 31*(6), 1163–1174.

Katare, B., Marshall, M. I., & Valdivia, C. B. (2021). Bend or break? Small business survival and strategies during the COVID-19 shock. *International Journal of Disaster Risk Reduction, 61*, 102332.

Kaushik, M., & Guleria, N. (2020). Employee relations and engagement during COVID-19. *Employee Relations, 3*(2), 1–11.

Kazancoglu, I., Ozbiltekin-Pala, M., Mangla, S. K., Kazancoglu, Y., & Jabeen, F. (2022). Role of flexibility, agility and responsiveness for sustainable supply chain resilience during COVID-19. *Journal of Cleaner Production, 362,* 132431.

Kharbat, F. F., Kannan, Y., Gleason, K., & Qasim, A. (2023). Corporate communication during the COVID-19 crisis in a multicultural environment: Culture and tweet impact. *Electronic Commerce Research.* https://doi.org/10.1007/s10660-023-09777-3

Kim, K., & Cho, K. T. (2021). A review of global collaboration on COVID-19 research during the pandemic in 2020. *Sustainability, 13*(14), 7618.

Kim, T. K., & Lane, S. R. (2013). Government health expenditure and public health outcomes: A comparative study among 17 countries and implications for US health care reform. *American International Journal of Contemporary Research, 3*(9), 8–13.

Kirk, L. E., & Mitchell, I. (2023). Has the COVID-19 pandemic unmasked the fragility of the Australian health care system? *The Medical Journal of Australia, 218*(10), 457–458.

Klein, K., Stolk, P., Tellner, P., Acha, V., Montagne, S., & Stöckert, I. (2022). Regulatory flexibilities and guidance for addressing the challenges of COVID-19 in the EU: What can we learn from company experiences? *Therapeutic Innovation & Regulatory Science, 56,* 366–377.

Klenert, D., Funke, F., Mattauch, L., & O'Callaghan, B. (2020). Five lessons from COVID-19 for advancing climate change mitigation. *Environmental and Resource Economics, 76,* 751–778.

Klobucista, C. (2022). *A guide to global COVID-19 vaccine efforts.* https://www.cfr.org/backgrounder/guide-global-COVID-19-vaccine-efforts

Knipsel, S. (2020). Tips for staying in with family and connecting with friends. *Futurity,* 23 March 2020. https://www.futurity.org/social-distancing-families-friends-psychology-2313782/

Koh, D. (2020). COVID-19 lockdowns throughout the world. *Occupational Medicine, 70*(5), 322–322.

Kong, Y., & Wu, R. (2023). Evolution of scholar networks during the COVID-19 outbreak. *Advances in Engineering Technology Research, 5*(1), 355–355.

Kourti, A., Stavridou, A., Panagouli, E., Psaltopoulou, T., Spiliopoulou, C., Tsolia, M., Sergentanis, T. N., & Tsitsika, A. (2023). Domestic violence during the COVID-19 pandemic: A systematic review. *Trauma, Violence, & Abuse, 24*(2), 719–745.

Krieger, R. (2019). *Public Policy, Health Care and Health Outcomes of the Poor in Advanced Democracies* (Doctoral dissertation). https://archive-ouverte.unige.ch/unige: 120768.

Kringos, D., Carinci, F., Barbazza, E., Bos, V., Gilmore, K., Groene, O., Gulácsi, L., Ivankovic, D., Jansen, T., Johnsen, S. P., de Lusignan, S., Mainz, J., Nuti, S., & Klazinga, N. (2020). Managing COVID-19 within and across health systems: Why we need performance intelligence to coordinate a global response. *Health Research Policy and Systems, 18,* 1–8.

Kuhfeld, M., Soland, J., Lewis, K., & Morton, E. (2022). The pandemic has had devastating impacts on learning. What will it take to help students catch up? https://www.brookings.edu/articles/the-pandemic-has-had-devastating-impacts-on-learning-what-will-it-take-to-help-students-catch-up/

Kumar, A. (2022). Customer retention in the covid era: Some insights for businesses. In Y. Azad, A. Sharma, & T. Sharma (Eds.), *Understanding interdisciplinary organizational flows* (pp. 29–36). Indu Book Services Pvt. Ltd.

Kumar, R. M. (2023). The many faces of grief: A systematic literature review of grief during the COVID-19 pandemic. *Illness, Crisis & Loss, 31*(1), 100–119.

Kumar, S., Basu, M., Ghosh, P., Ansari, A., & Ghosh, M. K. (2023). COVID-19: Clinical status of vaccine development to date. *British Journal of Clinical Pharmacology, 89*(1), 114–149.

Kurdin, A. A. (2020). Institutional continuum in the context of the pandemic. *Population and Economics, 4*(2), 39–42.

Kwok, F., Sharma, P., Gaur, S. S., & Ueno, A. (2019). Interactive effects of information exchange, relationship capital and environmental uncertainty on international joint venture (IJV) performance: An emerging markets perspective. *International Business Review, 28*(5), 101481.

LaBerge, L., O'Toole, C., Schneider, J., & Smaj, K. (2020). How COVID-19 has pushed companies over the technology tipping point—and transformed business forever? *McKinsey & Company,* 1–9. https://www.mckinsey.com/capabilities/strategy-and-corporate-finance/our-insights/.

Lachance, E. L. (2021). COVID-19 and its impact on volunteering: Moving towards virtual volunteering. *Leisure Sciences, 43*(1–2), 104–110.

Lagman, J. D. N. (2021). Vaccine nationalism: A predicament in ending the COVID-19 pandemic. *Journal of Public Health, 43*(2), e375–e376.

Lallie, H. S., Shepherd, L. A., Nurse, J. R., Erola, A., Epiphaniou, G., Maple, C., & Bellekens, X. (2021). Cyber security in the age of COVID-19: A timeline and analysis of cyber-crime and cyber-attacks during the pandemic. *Computers & Security, 105,* 102248.

Lee, A. (2020). Wuhan Novel coronavirus (COVID-19): Why global control is challenging? *Public Health, 179,* A1.

Lee, S. T. (2023). Vaccine diplomacy: Nation branding and China's COVID-19 soft power play. *Place Branding and Public Diplomacy, 19,* 64–78.

Lee, J. J., & Haupt, J. P. (2021). Scientific collaboration on COVID-19 amidst geopolitical tensions between the US and China. *The Journal of Higher Education, 92*(2), 303–329.

Leung, H. (2020). Why wearing a face mask is encouraged in Asia, but shunned in the US. *Time,* 12 March 2020, https://time.com/5799964/coronavirus-face-mask-asia-us/.

Leung, T. Y., Sharma, P., Adithipyangkul, P., & Hosie, P. (2020). Gender equity and public health outcomes: The COVID-19 experience. *Journal of Business Research, 116,* 193–198.

Li, D. (2022). The shift to online classes during the COVID-19 pandemic: Benefits, challenges, and required improvements from the students' perspective. *Electronic Journal of E-Learning, 20*(1), 1–18.

Libotte, G. B., Lobato, F. S., Platt, G. M., & Neto, A. J. S. (2020). Determination of an optimal control strategy for vaccine administration in COVID-19 pandemic treatment. *Computer Methods and Programs in Biomedicine, 196,* 105664.

Liu, Z., Guo, J., Zhong, W., & Gui, T. (2021). Multi-level governance, policy coordination and subnational responses to COVID-19: Comparing China and the US. *Journal of Comparative Policy Analysis: Research and Practice, 23*(2), 204–218.

Liu, Y., Lee, J. M., & Lee, C. (2020). The challenges and opportunities of a global health crisis: The management and business implications of COVID-19 from an Asian perspective. *Asian Business & Management, 19,* 277–297.

Liu, J., Shahab, Y., & Hoque, H. (2022). Government response measures and public trust during the COVID-19 pandemic: Evidence from around the world. *British Journal of Management, 33*(2), 571–602.

Lund, S., Madgavkar, A., Manyika, J., Smit, S., Ellingrud, E., & Robinson, O. (2021). The future of work after COVID-19. *McKinsey & Company,* 1–30. https://www.mckinsey.com/featured-insights/future-of-work/the-future-of-work-after-covid-19.

Lusardi, A., Hasler, A., & Yakoboski, P. J. (2021). Building up financial literacy and financial resilience. *Mind & Society, 20,* 181–187.

Luthra, S. (2021). The impact of covid-19 on consumer perception towards subscription based OTT platforms. *International Journal of Management (IJM), 12*(3), 537–549.

Maani, N., & Galea, S. (2020). COVID-19 and underinvestment in the public health infrastructure of the United States. *The Milbank Quarterly, 98*(2), 250–259.

MacIntyre, C. R. (2020). Global spread of COVID-19 and pandemic potential. *Global Biosecurity, 1*(3), 1–3.

Mahdi, O. R., & Nassar, I. A. (2021). The business model of sustainable competitive advantage through strategic leadership capabilities and knowledge management processes to overcome covid-19 pandemic. *Sustainability, 13*(17), 9891.

Mahmud, A., Ding, D., & Hasan, M. M. (2021). Corporate social responsibility: Business responses to coronavirus (COVID-19) pandemic. *SAGE Open, 11*(1), 2158244020988710.

Malik, M. A. (2022). Fragility and challenges of health systems in pandemic: Lessons from India's second wave of coronavirus disease 2019 (COVID-19). *Global Health Journal, 6*(1), 44–49.

Manguvo, A., & Mafuvadze, B. (2015). The impact of traditional and religious practices on the spread of Ebola in West Africa: Time for a strategic shift. *The Pan African Medical Journal, 22*(Supp 1), 9.

Mansour, H. (2022). How successful countries are in promoting digital transactions during COVID-19. *Journal of Economic Studies, 49*(3), 435–452.

Margherita, A., & Heikkilä, M. (2021). Business continuity in the COVID-19 emergency: A framework of actions undertaken by world-leading companies. *Business Horizons, 64*(5), 683–695.

Marhraoui, M. A. (2023). Digital skills for project managers: A systematic literature review. *Procedia Computer Science, 219,* 1591–1598.

Masonbrink, A. R., & Hurley, E. (2020). Advocating for children during the COVID-19 school closures. *Pediatrics, 146*(3), e20201440.

Mattera, M., Soto Gonzalez, F., Alba Ruiz-Morales, C., & Gava, L. (2021). Facing a global crisis-how sustainable business models helped firms overcome COVID. *Corporate Governance, 21*(6), 1100–1116.

Matusitz, J., & Musambira, G. (2013). Power distance, uncertainty avoidance, and technology: Analyzing Hofstede's dimensions and human development indicators. *Journal of Technology in Human Services, 31*(1), 42–60.

McLean, G., Kamil, J., Lee, B., Moore, P., Schulz, T. F., Muik, A., Sahin, U., Türeci, Ö, & Pather, S. (2022). The impact of evolving SARS-CoV-2 mutations and variants on COVID-19 vaccines. *mBio, 13*(2), e02979–21.

Mehdipanah, R. (2020). Housing as a determinant of COVID-19 inequities. *American Journal of Public Health, 110*(9), 1369–1370.

Memon, Z., Qureshi, S., & Memon, B. R. (2021). Assessing the role of quarantine and isolation as control strategies for COVID-19 outbreak: A case study. *Chaos, Solitons & Fractals, 144*, 110655.

Mertens, W., Pugliese, A., & Recker, J. (2017). Causality: Endogeneity biases and possible remedies. In W. Mertens (Ed.), *Quantitative data analysis* (pp. 99–134). Springer.

Miao, Q., Newman, A., Schwarz, G., & Xu, L. (2013). Participative leadership and the organizational commitment of civil servants in China: The mediating effects of trust in supervisor. *British Journal of Management, 24*(S1), S76–S92.

Mikołajczyk, K. (2022). Changes in the approach to employee development in organisations as a result of the COVID-19 pandemic. *European Journal of Training and Development, 46*(5/6), 544–562.

Minbaeva, D., Rabbiosi, L., & Stahl, G. K. (2018). Not walking the talk? How host country cultural orientations may buffer the damage of corporate values' misalignment in multinational corporations. *Journal of World Business, 53*(6), 880–895.

Minkov, M. (2018). A revision of Hofstede's model of national culture: Old evidence and new data from 56 countries. *Cross Cultural & Strategic Management, 25*(2), 231–256.

Mishra, V., Seyedzenouzi, G., Almohtadi, A., Chowdhury, T., Khashkhusha, A., Axiaq, A., Wong, W. Y. E., & Harky, A. (2021). Health inequalities during COVID-19 and their effects on morbidity and mortality. *Journal of Healthcare Leadership, 13*, 19–26.

Mittal, A., Mantri, A., Tandon, U., & Dwivedi, Y. K. (2022). A unified perspective on the adoption of online teaching in higher education during the COVID-19 pandemic. *Information Discovery and Delivery, 50*(2), 117–132.

Modgil, S., Singh, R. K., & Hannibal, C. (2022). Artificial intelligence for supply chain resilience: Learning from covid-19. *The International Journal of Logistics Management, 33*(4), 1246–1268.

Mohd-Dom, T. N., Lim, K. X., Rani, H., & Yew, H. Z. (2022). Malaysian dental deans' consensus on impact of COVID-19 and recommendations for sustaining quality dental education. *Frontiers in Education, 7*, 926376.

Monni, S., & Spaventa, A. (2013). Beyond GDP and HDI: Shifting the focus from paradigms to politics. *Development, 56*(2), 227–231.

Moosavi, J., Fathollahi-Fard, A. M., & Dulebenets, M. A. (2022). Supply chain disruption during the COVID-19 pandemic: Recognizing potential disruption management strategies. *International Journal of Disaster Risk Reduction, 75*, 102983.

Mukherjee, W. (2020). Covid-19 fear: Electronics brands Samsung, Apple let offline stores sell online. The Economic Times, India, 18 April 2020.

Narayanamurthy, G., & Tortorella, G. (2021). Impact of COVID-19 outbreak on employee performance–moderating role of industry 4.0 base technologies. *International Journal of Production Economics, 234*, 108075.

Natoli, R., & Zuhair, S. (2011). Measuring progress: A comparison of the GDP, HDI, GS and the RIE. *Social Indicators Research, 103*, 33–56.

Noar, S. M., & Austin, L. (2020). (Mis)communicating about COVID-19: Insights from health and crisis communication. *Health Communication, 35*(14), 1735–1739.

North, D. C. (1991). Institutions. *Journal of Economic Perspectives, 5*(1), 97–112.

OECD. (2020a). Transparency, communication and trust: The role of public communication in responding to the wave of disinformation about the new Coronavirus. *OECD Policy Responses to Coronavirus (COVID-19)*. https://www.oecd.org/coronavirus/policy-responses/transparency-communication-and-trust-the-role-of-public-communication-in-responding-to-the-wave-of-disinformation-about-the-new-coronavirus-bef7ad6e/.

OECD. (2020b). Digital transformation in the age of COVID-19: Building resilience and bridging divides, digital economy outlook 2020 supplement, *OECD*, Paris.

Oney, M. (2012). *An analysis of the relationship between health expenditure and health outcomes* (Doctoral dissertation). https://digital.maag.ysu.edu/xmlui/handle/1989/10511.

Oxfam (2021). The inequality virus. *Oxfam International.* https://oxfamilibrary.openrepository.com

Ozdemir, D., Sharma, M., Dhir, A., & Daim, T. (2022). Supply chain resilience during the COVID-19 pandemic. *Technology in Society, 68*, 101847.

Pacheco, G., van der Westhuizen, D. W., Ghobadian, A., Webber, D. J., & O'Regan, N. (2016). The changing influence of societal culture on job satisfaction across Europe. *British Journal of Management, 27*(3), 606–627.

Panchal, N., Saunders, H., Rudowitz, R., & Cox, C. (2023). *The implications of COVID-19 for mental health and substance use* (20 March 2023). https://www.kff.org/mental-health/issue-brief/the-implications-of-COVID-19-for-mental-health-and-substance-use.

Panwar, R., Pinkse, J., & De Marchi, V. (2022). The future of global supply chains in a post-COVID-19 world. *California Management Review, 64*(2), 5–23.

Papadopoulos, R. (2022). The covid-19 pandemic and cultural competence: Global implications for managers, nurses and healthcare workers during major health disasters and emergencies. *Journal of Nursing Management, 30*(7), 2451–2452.

Patel, J. A., Nielsen, F. B. H., Badiani, A. A., Assi, S., Unadkat, V. A., Patel, B., Ravindrane, R., & Wardle, H. (2020a). Poverty, inequality and COVID-19: The forgotten vulnerable. *Public Health, 183*, 110–111.

Patel, A., Patel, S., Fulzele, P., Mohod, S., & Chhabra, K. G. (2020b). Quarantine an effective mode for control of the spread of COVID19? A review. *Journal of Family Medicine and Primary Care, 9*(8), 3867.

Patterson, R. N. (2020). How to reform healthcare after Covid-19. *The Bulwark*, 20 April 2020. https://thebulwark.com/how-to-reform-healthcare-in-the-wake-of-covid-19/.

Peretz, H., Fried, Y., & Levi, A. (2018). Flexible work arrangements, national culture, organisational characteristics, and organisational outcomes: A study across 21 countries. *Human Resource Management Journal, 28*(1), 182–200.

Qato, D. (2020). Our public health infrastructure is losing a fight with capitalism. *Jacobin Magazine*, 20 March 2020. https://www.jacobinmag.com/2020/03/coronavirus-public-health-infrastructure-capitalism-epidemiology.

Qin, Y. S., & Men, L. R. (2023). Exploring the impact of internal communication on employee psychological well-being during the COVID-19 pandemic: The mediating role of employee organizational trust. *International Journal of Business Communication, 60*(4), 1197–1219.

Rabiul, M. K., Promsivapallop, P., Al Karim, R., Islam, M. A., & Patwary, A. K. (2022). Fostering quality customer service during covid-19: The role of managers' Oral language, employee work engagement, and employee resilience. *Journal of Hospitality and Tourism Management, 53*, 50–60.

Rahman, M. K., Gazi, M. A. I., Bhuiyan, M. A., & Rahaman, M. A. (2021). Effect of COVID-19 pandemic on tourist travel risk and management perceptions. *PLoS ONE*, *16*(9), e0256486.

Raimo, N., Rella, A., Vitolla, F., Sánchez-Vicente, M. I., & García-Sánchez, I. M. (2021). Corporate social responsibility in the COVID-19 pandemic period: A traditional way to address new social issues. *Sustainability*, *13*(12), 6561.

Ramsay, S. (2020). Let's not return to business as usual: Integrating environmental and social wellbeing through hybrid business models post COVID-19. *International Social Work*, *63*(6), 798–802.

Rana, R. H., Alam, K., & Gow, J. (2020). Health expenditure and gross domestic product: Causality analysis by income level. *International Journal of Health Economics and Management*, *20*, 55–77.

Rathod, S., Rathod, P., & Phiri, P. (2020). Impact of culture on response to COVID 19. *BMJ*, https://doi.org/10.1136/bmj.m1556.

Reddin, K., Bang, H., & Miles, L. (2021). Evaluating simulations as preparation for health crises like COVID-19: Insights on incorporating simulation exercises for effective response. *International Journal of Disaster Risk Reduction*, *59*, 102245.

Roozen, G. V., Roukens, A. H., & Roestenberg, M. (2022). COVID-19 vaccine dose sparing: Strategies to improve vaccine equity and pandemic preparedness. *The Lancet Global Health*, *10*(4), e570–e573.

Ros, F., Kush, R., Friedman, C., Gil Zorzo, E., Rivero Corte, P., Rubin, J. C., Sanchez, B., Stocco, P., & Van Houweling, D. (2021). Addressing the Covid-19 pandemic and future public health challenges through global collaboration and a data-driven systems approach. *Learning Health Systems*, *5*(1), e10253.

Rydland, H. T., Friedman, J., Stringhini, S., Link, B. G., & Eikemo, T. A. (2022). The radically unequal distribution of covid-19 vaccinations: A predictable yet avoidable symptom of the fundamental causes of inequality. *Humanities and Social Sciences Communications*, *9*, 61.

Ryu, S., & Cho, D. (2022). The show must go on? The entertainment industry during (and after) COVID-19. *Media, Culture & Society*, *44*(3), 591–600.

Saltzman, L. Y., Lesen, A. E., Henry, V., Hansel, T. C., & Bordnick, P. S. (2021). COVID-19 mental health disparities. *Health Security*, *19*(S1), S-5.

Sangster Jokić, C. A., & Jokić-Begić, N. (2022). Occupational disruption during the COVID-19 pandemic: Exploring changes to daily routines and their potential impact on mental health. *Journal of Occupational Science*, *29*(3), 336–351.

Santomauro, D. F., Herrera, A. M. M., Shadid, J., Zheng, P., Ashbaugh, C., Pigott, D., Hay, S. I., Vos, T., Murray, C. J. L., Whiteford, H. A., Ferrari, A. J., Abbafati, C., Adolph, C., Amlag, J., Bang-Jensen, B. L., Bertolacci, G. J., Bloom, S., Castellano, R., Castro, E., …, Zigler, B. (2021). Global prevalence and burden of depressive and anxiety disorders in 204 countries and territories in 2020 due to the COVID-19 pandemic. *The Lancet*, *398*(10312), 1700–1712.

Sauer, M. A., Truelove, S., Gerste, A. K., & Limaye, R. J. (2021). A failure to communicate? How public messaging has strained the COVID-19 response in the United States. *Health Security*, *19*(1), 65–74.

Scandurra, C., Bochicchio, V., Dolce, P., Valerio, P., Muzii, B., & Maldonato, N. M. (2023). Why people were less compliant with public health regulations during the second wave of the covid-19 outbreak: The role of trust in governmental organizations, future anxiety, fatigue, and covid-19 risk perception. *Current Psychology*, *42*, 7403–7413.

Scholl, W., & Schermuly, C. C. (2020). The impact of culture on corruption, gross domestic product, and human development. *Journal of Business Ethics*, *162*(1), 171–189.

Schuitevoerder, R. (2023). *How the covid pandemic has helped the EdTech industry grow.* https://www.thecfigroup.com/news/how-the-covid-pandemic-has-helped-the-edtech-industry-grow/.

Self, S., & Grabowski, R. (2003). How effective is public health expenditure in improving overall health? A cross–country analysis. *Applied Economics, 35*(7), 835–845.

Shah, A., & Coiado, O. C. (2023). COVID-19 vaccine and booster hesitation around the world: A literature review. *Frontiers in Medicine, 9,* 1054557.

Sharif, A., Aloui, C., & Yarovaya, L. (2020). COVID-19 pandemic, oil prices, stock market, geopolitical risk and policy uncertainty nexus in the US economy: Fresh evidence from the wavelet-based approach. *International Review of Financial Analysis, 70,* 101496.

Sharma, A., Borah, S. B., & Moses, A. C. (2021). Responses to COVID-19: The role of governance, healthcare infrastructure, and learning from past pandemics. *Journal of Business Research, 122,* 597–607.

Sharma, G. D., Kraus, S., Srivastava, M., Chopra, R., & Kallmuenzer, A. (2022). The changing role of innovation for crisis management in times of COVID-19: An integrative literature review. *Journal of Innovation & Knowledge, 7*(4), 100281.

Sharma, P., Leung, T. Y., Kingshott, R. P. J., Davcik, N., & Cardinali, S. (2020). Managing uncertainty during a global pandemic: An international business perspective. *Journal of Business Research, 116,* 188–192.

Sharma, M., Singh, A., & Daim, T. (2023). Exploring cloud computing adoption: COVID era in academic institutions. *Technological Forecasting and Social Change, 193,* 122613.

Sharma, O., Sultan, A. A., Ding, H., & Triggle, C. R. (2020). A review of the progress and challenges of developing a vaccine for COVID-19. *Frontiers in Immunology, 11,* 585354.

Sharun, K., & Dhama, K. (2021). India's role in COVID-19 vaccine diplomacy. *Journal of Travel Medicine, 28*(7), taab064.

Shehzad, K., Xiaoxing, L., Arif, M., Rehman, K. U., & Ilyas, M. (2020). Investigating the psychology of financial markets during COVID-19 era: A case study of the US and European markets. *Frontiers in Psychology, 11,* 1924.

Sheikh, Z., Ghaffar, A., Islam, T., & Sheikh, A. A. (2023). Consumers' acceptance of social commerce during COVID-19 lockdown. *Journal of Global Scholars of Marketing Science, 33*(2), 210–230.

Sheldon, D. (2021). Policing the pandemic: Maintaining compliance and legitimacy during COVID-19. *King's Law Journal, 32*(1), 14–25.

Shereen, M. A., Khan, S., Kazmi, A., Bashir, N., & Siddique, R. (2020). COVID-19 infection: Emergence, transmission, and characteristics of human coronaviruses. *Journal of Advanced Research, 24,* 91–98.

Silliman Cohen, R. I., & Bosk, E. A. (2020). Vulnerable youth and the COVID-19 pandemic. *Pediatrics, 146*(1), e20201306.

Simonsen, L., & Viboud, C. (2021). A comprehensive look at the COVID-19 pandemic death toll. *Elife, 10,* e71974.

Simpeh, F., & Amoah, C. (2022). COVID-19 guidelines incorporated in the health and safety management policies of construction firms. *Journal of Engineering, Design and Technology, 20*(1), 6–23.

Singh, V., Shirazi, H., & Turetken, J. (2022). COVID-19 and gender disparities: Labour market outcomes. *Research in Economics, 76*(3), 206–217.

Singh, S., Yadav, B., & Batheri, R. (2023). Industry 4.0: Meeting the challenges of demand sensing in the automotive industry. *IEEE Engineering Management Review*. https://doi.org/10.1109/EMR.2023.3292331

Sirkeci, I., & Yüceşahin, M. (2020). Coronavirus and migration: Analysis of human mobility and the spread of covid-19. *Migration Letters*, *17*(2), 379–398.

Smith, P. B. (1992). Organizational behaviour and national cultures. *British Journal of Management*, *3*(1), 39–51.

Smith, P. B., Dugan, S., & Trompenaars, F. (1996). National culture and the values of organizational employees: A dimensional analysis across 43 nations. *Journal of Cross-Cultural Psychology*, *27*(2), 231–264.

Sodhi, M. S., Tang, C. S., & Willenson, E. T. (2023). Research opportunities in preparing supply chains of essential goods for future pandemics. *International Journal of Production Research*, *61*(8), 2416–2431.

Sparke, M., & Levy, O. (2022). Competing responses to global inequalities in access to COVID vaccines: Vaccine diplomacy and vaccine charity versus vaccine liberty. *Clinical Infectious Diseases*, *75*(S1), S86–S92.

Spieske, A., & Birkel, H. (2021). Improving supply chain resilience through industry 4.0: A systematic literature review under the impressions of the COVID-19 pandemic. *Computers & Industrial Engineering*, *158*, 107452.

Stann, E. (2020). How culture affects the spread of pandemics like Covid-19. *Futurity*, 27 March 2020. https://www.futurity.org/covid-19-culture-history-2318752/.

Statista. (2023). Impact of the coronavirus pandemic on the global economy - Statistics & Facts. https://www.statista.com/topics/6139/covid-19-impact-on-the-global-economy/.

Stavrou, E., & Kilaniotis, C. (2010). Flexible work and turnover: An empirical investigation across cultures. *British Journal of Management*, *21*(2), 541–554.

Stiglitz, J. E. (2021). The proper role of government in the market economy: The case of the post-COVID recovery. *Journal of Government and Economics*, *1*, 100004.

Stobart, A., & Duckett, S. (2022). Australia's response to COVID-19. *Health Economics, Policy and Law*, *17*(1), 95–106.

Strusani, D., & Houngbonon, G. V. (2020). What COVID-19 means for digital infrastructure in emerging markets. *International Finance Corporation*, Note 83, May 2020. https://www.ifc.org/thoughtleadership.

Stuart, M., Spencer, D. A., McLachlan, C. J., & Forde, C. (2021). COVID-19 and the uncertain future of HRM: Furlough, job retention and reform. *Human Resource Management Journal*, *31*(4), 904–917.

Sun, L., Small, G., Huang, Y. H., & Ger, T. B. (2022). Financial shocks, financial stress and financial resilience of Australian households during COVID-19. *Sustainability*, *14*(7), 3736.

Tang, R., Jiang, J., Zhang, Y., & Luo, J. (2023). Open government data (OGD) sites and the sharing of country-specific real-time pandemic information: An investigation into COVID-19 datasets available on worldwide OGDs. *Information Processing & Management*, *60*(6), 103489.

Tang, L., & Koveos, P. E. (2008). A framework to update Hofstede's cultural value indices: Economic dynamics and institutional stability. *Journal of International Business Studies*, *39*, 1045–1063.

Tarkar, P. (2020). Impact of COVID-19 pandemic on education system. *International Journal of Advanced Science and Technology*, *29*(9), 3812–3814.

Taylor, A., Fram, A., Kellman, L., & Superville, D. (2020). Trump signs $2.2T stimulus after swift congressional votes. *Associated Press*, 28 March 2020. https://apnews.com/article/donald-trump-financial-markets-ap-top-news-bills-virus-outbreak-2099a53bb8adf2def7ee7329ea322f9d.

The Lancet Public Health (2022). COVID-19 pandemic: What's next for public health? *Lancet Public Health*, 7(5), e391. https://doi.org/10.1016/S2468-2667(22)00095-0.

Thompson, E. R., & Phua, F. T. (2005). Are national cultural traits applicable to senior firm managers? *British Journal of Management*, 16(1), 59–68.

Thye, A. Y. K., Tan, L. T. H., Law, J. W. F., & Letchumanan, V. (2021). COVID-19 booster vaccines administration in different countries. *Progress in Microbes & Molecular Biology*, 4(1), a0000256.

Tran, A., & Witek, T. J. Jr. (2021). The emergency use authorization of pharmaceuticals: History and utility during the COVID-19 pandemic. *Pharmaceutical Medicine*, 35, 203–213.

Tsamakis, K., Tsiptsios, D., Ouranidis, A., Mueller, C., Schizas, D., Terniotis, C., Nikolakakis, N., Tyros, G., Kympouropoulos, S., Lazaris, A., Spandidos, D.A., Smyrnis, N., & Rizos, E. (2021). COVID-19 and its consequences on mental health. *Experimental and Therapeutic Medicine*, 21(3), 244.

Tulaskar, R., & Turunen, M. (2022). What students want? Experiences, challenges, and engagement during emergency remote learning amidst COVID-19 crisis. *Education and Information Technologies*, 27(1), 551–587.

Tulenko, K., & Vervoort, D. (2020). Cracks in the system: The effects of the coronavirus pandemic on public health systems. *The American Review of Public Administration*, 50(6–7), 455–466.

Tzenios, N., Chahine, M., & Tazanios, M. (2023). Better strategies for coronavirus (COVID-19) vaccination. *Special Journal of the Medical Academy and Other Life Sciences.*, 1(2).

Uddin, S., Ahmed, M. S., & Shahadat, K. (2023). Supply chain accountability, COVID-19, and violations of workers' rights in the global clothing supply chain. *Supply Chain Management*, 28(5), 859–873.

UNDP. (2020). *Global human development indicators*. United Nations Development Programme Human Development Reports.

UNESCO. (2020). *COVID-19 educational disruption and response*. United Nations Educational, Scientific and Cultural Organization. https://en.unesco.org/covid19.

United Nation. (2020). *Everyone included: Social impact of covid-19*. Department of Economic and Social Affairs, United Nations.

Vaiman, V., Cascio, W. F., Collings, D. G., & Swider, B. W. (2021). The shifting boundaries of talent management. *Human Resource Management*, 60(2), 253–257.

Verma, A., Venkatesan, M., Kumar, M., & Verma, J. (2023). The future of work post covid-19: Key perceived HR implications of hybrid workplaces in India. *Journal of Management Development*, 42(1), 13–28.

Versey, H. S. (2021). The impending eviction cliff: Housing insecurity during COVID-19. *American Journal of Public Health*, 111(8), 1423–1427.

Victor, G. S., & Ahmed, S. (2019). The importance of culture in managing mental health response to pandemics. In Huremović D. (Ed.), *Psychiatry of pandemics* (pp. 55–64). Springer. https://doi.org/10.1007/978-3-030-15346-5_5.

Villarreal, A., & Yu, W. H. (2022). Research note: Gender differences in employment during the COVID-19 epidemic. *Demography*, 59(1), 13–26.

Viner, R. M., Russell, S. J., Croker, H., Packer, J., Ward, J., Stansfield, C., Mytton, O., Bonell, C., & Booy, R. (2020). School closure and management practices during coronavirus outbreaks including COVID-19: A rapid systematic review. *The Lancet Child & Adolescent Health*, 4(5), 397–404.

Vizheh, M., Qorbani, M., Arzaghi, S. M., Muhidin, S., Javanmard, Z., & Esmaeili, M. (2020). The mental health of healthcare workers in the COVID-19 pandemic: A systematic review. *Journal of Diabetes & Metabolic Disorders*, 19, 1967–1978.

Wang, J., Cui, M., & Chang, L. (2023). Evaluating economic recovery by measuring the COVID-19 spillover impact on business practices: Evidence from Asian markets intermediaries. *Economic Change and Restructuring*, 56, 1629–1650.

Wang, S., Kamerāde, D., Bessa, I., Burchell, B., Gifford, J., Green, M., & Rubery, J. (2022b). The impact of reduced working hours and furlough policies on workers' mental health at the onset of COVID-19 pandemic: A longitudinal study. *Journal of Social Policy*, 1–25. 10.1017/S0047279422000599

Wang, X., Wong, Y. D., Qi, G., & Yuen, K. F. (2021). Contactless channel for shopping and delivery in the context of social distancing in response to COVID-19 pandemic. *Electronic Commerce Research and Applications*, 48, 101075.

Wang, J., Zhu, H., Lai, X., Zhang, H., Huang, Y., Feng, H., Lyu, Y., Jing, R., Guo, J., & Fang, H. (2022a). From COVID-19 vaccination intention to actual vaccine uptake: A longitudinal study among Chinese adults after six months of a national vaccination campaign. *Expert Review of Vaccines*, 21(3), 385–395.

Wardana, L. W., Indrawati, A., Maula, F. I., Mahendra, A. M., Fatihin, M. K., Rahma, A., Nafisa, A., Putri, A. A., & Narmaditya, B. S. (2023). Do digital literacy and business sustainability matter for creative economy? The role of entrepreneurial attitude. *Heliyon*, 9, e12763.

Warne, D. J., Ebert, A., Drovandi, C., Hu, W., Mira, A., & Mengersen, K. (2020). Hindsight is 2020 vision: A characterisation of the global response to the COVID-19 pandemic. *BMC Public Health*, 20, 1868.

WEF. (2022). What COVID-19 taught us about collaboration – 7 lessons from the frontline. *World Economic Forum*, 21 April 2022.

Wei, Y., Guan, J., Ning, X., Li, Y., Wei, L., Shen, S., Zhang, R., Zhao, Y., Shen, H., & Chen, F. (2022). Global COVID-19 pandemic waves: Limited lessons learned worldwide over the past year. *Engineering*, 13, 91–98.

Wetherall, K., Cleare, S., McClelland, H., Melson, A.J., Niedzwiedz, C.L., O'Carroll, R.E., O'Connor, D.B., Platt, S., Scowcroft, E., Watson, B., Zortea, T. Ferguson, E., Robb, K.A., & O'Connor, R. (2022). Mental health and well-being during the second wave of COVID-19: Longitudinal analyses of the UK COVID-19 mental health and wellbeing study (UK COVID-MH). *BJPsych Open*, 8(4), e103.

WHO. (2020). WHO director-general's opening remarks at the media briefing on COVID-19. *World Health Organization*, 11 March 2020.

WHO. (2022). The impact of COVID-19 on mental health cannot be made light of. *World Health Organization*, 16 June 2022. https://www.who.int/news-room/feature-stories/detail/the-impact-of-covid-19-on-mental-health-cannot-be-made-light-of.

WHO. (2023). Coronavirus disease (COVID-19) weekly epidemiological updates and monthly operational updates. *World Health Organization*. https://www.who.int/emergencies/diseases/novel-coronavirus-2019/situation-reports

Williamson, B., Macgilchrist, F., & Potter, J. (2021). Covid-19 controversies and critical research in digital education. *Learning, Media and Technology, 46*(2), 117–127.

Williams, C. Y., Townson, A. T., Kapur, M., Ferreira, A. F., Nunn, R., Galante, J., Phillips, V., Gentry, S., & Usher-Smith, J. A. (2021). Interventions to reduce social isolation and loneliness during COVID-19 physical distancing measures: A rapid systematic review. *PLoS ONE, 16*(2), e0247139.

Wittenberg-Cox, A. (2020). What do countries with the Best coronavirus responses have in common? Women leadership. *Forbes Magazine*, 13 April 2020. https://www.forbes.com/sites/avivahwittenbergcox/2020/04/13/what-do-countries-with-the-best-coronavirus-reponses-have-in-common-women-leaders/?sh=25512d953dec

Wong, K. F. E., & Cheng, C. (2020). The turnover intention–behaviour link: A culture-moderated meta-analysis. *Journal of Management Studies, 57*(6), 1174–1216.

Wong, A., Olusanya, O., Parulekar, P., & Highfield, J. (2021). Staff wellbeing in times of COVID-19. *Journal of the Intensive Care Society, 22*(4), 328–334.

World Bank. (2020). *World Bank Open Data*, https://data.worldbank.org/.

World Bank. (2022). COVID-19 Drives Global Surge in use of Digital Payments. *World Bank Press Release* (29 June 2022). https://www.worldbank.org/en/news/press-release/2022/06/29/covid-19-drives-global-surge-in-use-of-digital-payments

World Bank. (2023). *World Development Report 2022: Finance for an Equitable Recovery*. https://www.worldbank.org/en/publication/wdr2022

Worldometer. (2020). https://www.worldometers.info/coronavirus.

Wursten, H. (2020). There is a system in the madness. The 7 mental images of national culture and the corona virus. *Journal of Intercultural Management and Ethics, 3*(1), 7–17.

Xin, M., Luo, S., She, R., Yu, Y., Li, L., Wang, S., Ma, L., Tao, F., Zhang, J., Zhao, J., Li, L., Hu, D., Zhang, G., Gu, J., Lin, D., Wang, H., Cai, Y. Wang, Z., You, H., …, Lau, T.F. (2020). Negative cognitive and psychological correlates of mandatory quarantine during the initial COVID-19 outbreak in China. *American Psychologist, 75*(5), 607–617.

Yi, F., Woo, J. J., & Zhang, Q. (2023). Community resilience and COVID-19: A fuzzy-set qualitative comparative analysis of resilience attributes in 16 countries. *International Journal of Environmental Research and Public Health, 20*(1), 474.

Yoch, M., & Sirull, R. (2021). New global burden of disease analyses show depression and anxiety among the top causes of health loss worldwide, and a significant increase due to the COVID-19 pandemic. The Institute for Health Metrics and Evaluation (8 October 2021). https://www.healthdata.org/news-events/insights-blog/acting-data/new-global-burden-disease-analyses-show-depression-and

Yue, C. A., & Walden, J. (2023). Guiding employees through the COVID-19 pandemic: An exploration of the impact of transparent communication and change appraisals. *Journal of Contingencies and Crisis Management, 31*(2), 198–211.

Zaki, B. L., Nicoli, F., Wayenberg, E., & Verschuere, B. (2022). Contagious inequality: Economic disparities and excess mortality during the COVID-19 pandemic. *Policy and Society, 41*(2), 199–216.

Zhai, Y., & Du, X. (2020). Loss and grief amidst COVID-19: A path to adaptation and resilience. *Brain, Behavior, and Immunity, 87*, 80–81.

Zhang, J., & Wang, Y. (2022). Effectiveness of corporate social responsibility activities in the COVID-19 pandemic. *Journal of Product & Brand Management, 31*(7), 1063–1076.

Appendix-I: Country-wise first COVID-19 cases

Country	First case date	Days since outbreak (1 December 2019)	First case description
Caribbeans			
Dominican Republic	2020-03-01	91	A man from Italy
Jamaica	2020-03-11	101	A female who arrived from the United Kingdom
Saint Vincent and the Grenadines	2020-03-11	101	The patient who had a travel history in the UK and Barbados
Cayman Islands	2020-03-12	102	An Italian man who was transferred from the cruise ship Costa Luminosa to a hospital in the Cayman Islands
Trinidad and Tobago	2020-03-12	102	A man who had a travel history in Switzerland
Cuba	2020-03-12	102	Three Italian tourists
Antigua and Barbuda	2020-03-13	103	A female from the UK
Saint Lucia	2020-03-13	103	A female with a travel history from the UK
Bahamas	2020-03-16	106	Exposure was unknown as the first patient was a female resident who did not have relevant travel history
Barbados	2020-03-17	107	A visitor who arrived from the US and a female Barbadian who returned from the US
Montserrat	2020-03-18	108	An individual who had a travel history in London and Antigua
Haiti	2020-03-20	110	A Haitian who returned from Paris and a Belgian volunteering in a Port-au-Prince orphanage
Grenada	2020-03-22	112	A female who returned from the UK
Dominica	2020-03-22	112	A man who returned from the UK

(*Continued*)

Country	First case date	Days since outbreak (1 December 2019)	First case description
Turks and Caicos Islands	2020-03-23	113	An individual who had no travel history
Anguilla	2020-03-24	114	An American woman and a resident of Anguilla with whom the American female had contact
Saint Kitts and Nevis	2020-03-24	114	Male and female nationals who returned from New York City
Central America			
Costa Rica	2020-03-06	96	An American woman tourist from New York (USA)
Panama	2020-03-10	100	An individual who arrived from Spain
Honduras	2020-03-11	101	A pregnant female who returned from Spain and a Honduran female who returned from Switzerland
Guatemala	2020-03-14	104	A Guatemalan man who returned from Italy
Nicaragua	2020-03-19	109	A man who returned from Panama
El Salvador	2020-03-19	109	A male who was in Italy
Belize	2020-03-23	113	A Belizean female who returned from LA, USA
North America			
The United States	2020-01-21	51	A Washington state resident who returned from Wuhan
Canada	2020-01-26	56	An individual who returned from Wuhan
Mexico	2020-02-28	89	Mexicans who returned from Bergamo (Italy)
Greenland	2020-03-16	106	The first patient lived in the capital, Nuuk
Bermuda	2020-03-18	108	An individual who had a travel history in the UK and US
South America			
Brazil	2020-02-26	87	A Brazilian who returned from Lombardy (Italy)
Ecuador	2020-03-01	91	A woman and an Ecuadorian citizen who resided in Spain
Chile	2020-03-03	93	A Chilean who had a travel history in Southeast Asia and Europe
Argentina	2020-03-03	93	A man who arrived from Milan (Italy)
Peru	2020-03-06	96	A Peruvian who returned from travels in France, Spain, and the Czech Republic
Colombia	2020-03-06	96	A female who had a travel history in Milan (Italy)
Paraguay	2020-03-08	98	A man who arrived from Guayaquil (Ecuador)
Bolivia	2020-03-11	101	Females who had a travel history in Italy

(Continued)

Country	First case date	Days since outbreak (1 December 2019)	First case description
Guyana	2020-03-12	102	A female who had a travel history in New York
Suriname	2020-03-13	103	An individual who arrived from the Netherlands
Uruguay	2020-03-13	103	People who arrived from Milan (Italy)
Venezuela	2020-03-14	104	Two tourists from Spain
Falkland Islands	2020-04-03	124	A British serviceperson came from the Mount Pleasant base (UK military base)
Central Africa			
Cameroon	2020-03-06	96	A French national arriving at Cameron
Democratic Republic of Congo	2020-03-11	101	A Congolese citizen who returned from France
Gabon	2020-03-12	102	A Gabonese man who returned from France
Equatorial Guinea	2020-03-15	105	A female who returned from Madrid
Central African Republic	2020-03-15	105	An Italian man who had a travel history in Milan (Italy)
Congo	2020-03-15	105	A man who returned from Paris (France)
Chad	2020-03-19	109	A Moroccan passenger flew from Douala
Angola	2020-03-20	110	An individual who returned from Portugal
Sao Tome and Principe	2020-04-06	127	
East Africa			
Kenya	2020-03-13	103	A Kenyan female who returned from the US via London
Sudan	2020-03-13	103	A man who visited the United Arab Emirates
Ethiopia	2020-03-13	103	The first patient was a Japanese citizen
Seychelles	2020-03-14	104	The patients were in contact with someone in Italy
Rwanda	2020-03-14	104	An Indian citizen who arrived from Mumbai (India)
Somalia	2020-03-16	106	A Somali citizen who returned from China
Tanzania	2020-03-16	106	A Tanzanian who returned from Belgium
Mauritius	2020-03-18	108	Mauritian nationals, two of whom were employees on a cruise ship while one returned from the UK
Djibouti	2020-03-18	108	A member of the Spanish Special Forces who arrived for Operation Atalanta
Zambia	2020-03-18	108	A couple who had a travel history in France

(Continued)

Country	First case date	Days since outbreak (1 December 2019)	First case description
Zimbabwe	2020-03-20	110	A male resident who returned from the UK via South Africa
Madagascar	2020-03-20	110	Two Malagasy citizens who returned from France and a Malagasy citizen who returned from Mauritius
Eritrea	2020-03-21	111	An Eritrean national who returned from Norway
Mozambique	2020-03-22	112	A man who returned from the UK
Uganda	2020-03-22	112	A male who had a travel history in Dubai
Burundi	2020-03-31	121	Burundi nationals who returned from Rwanda and Dubai
Malawi	2020-04-02	123	A Malawian of Asian origin who returned from India and her relative and their housemaid
South Sudan	2020-04-05	126	A United Nations worker from the Netherlands via Ethiopia
Comoros	2020-04-30	151	A man in contact with a Franco-Comorian national
Northern Africa			
Egypt	2020-02-14	75	A Chinese national
Algeria	2020-02-25	86	An Italian man
Morocco	2020-03-02	92	A Moroccan expatriate residing in Bergamo (Italy)
Tunisia	2020-03-02	92	A Tunisian man who returned from Italy
Libya	2020-03-24	114	A man who returned from Saudi Arabia
Southern Africa			
South Africa	2020-03-05	95	A male citizen who returned from Italy
Namibia	2020-03-14	104	A Romanian couple who arrived from Spain via Doha
Eswatini	2020-03-14	104	A female who returned from the US and Lesotho
Botswana	2020-03-30	120	Citizens and residents (two males and one female) who had a travel history in high-risk countries (UK and Thailand)
Lesotho	2020-05-13	164	An individual who had a travel history in the Middle East
West Africa			
Nigeria	2020-02-28	89	An Italian citizen who arrived from Milan (Italy)
Senegal	2020-03-02	92	A man from France
Togo	2020-03-06	96	A Togolese woman who returned from a trip in Germany, France, Turkey, and Nenin
Burkina Faso	2020-03-10	100	A couple with a wife who returned from France

(Continued)

Country	First case date	Days since outbreak (1 December 2019)	First case description
Cote d'Ivoire	2020-03-11	101	An Ivorian who returned from Italy
Ghana	2020-03-12	102	One individual from Norway and one individual from Turkey
Guinea	2020-03-13	103	A Belgian national who worked in the EU delegation in Guinea
Mauritania	2020-03-14	104	A citizen of a European country
Benin	2020-03-16	106	An individual from Burkina Faso who had a travel history in Belgium
Liberia	2020-03-16	106	A government official who returned from Switzerland
Gambia	2020-03-17	107	A female who returned from the UK
Cape Verde	2020-03-20	110	A foreigner from the UK
Niger	2020-03-20	110	A man from Nigeria who had a travel history in Lome, Accra, Abidjan, and Ouagadougou
Mali	2020-03-25	115	Malian nationals who returned from France
Guinea-Bissau	2020-03-25	115	A Congolese UN employee and an Indian citizen
Sierra Leone	2020-03-31	121	A man who had a travel history in France
Central Asia			
Kazakhstan	2020-03-13	103	Two Kazakh citizens who returned from Germany
Uzbekistan	2020-03-15	105	An Uzbek citizen who returned from France
Kyrgyzstan	2020-03-18	108	A citizen who returned from Saudi Arabia
Tajikistan	2020-04-30	151	Fifteen confirmed cases including ten cases in Khujand and five in Dushanbe
East Asia			
China	2019-12-01	0	
Japan	2020-01-15	45	A resident who returned from Wuhan China
South Korea	2020-01-20	50	A female Chinese national residing in Wuhan (China)
Taiwan	2020-01-21	51	A female who returned from Wuhan
Mongolia	2020-03-10	100	A French national who arrived via a flight from Moscow
South Asia			
Nepal	2020-01-23	53	A man who returned from China
Sri Lanka	2020-01-27	57	A Chinese woman tourist from China
India	2020-01-30	60	Students who returned from Wuhan
Afghanistan	2020-02-24	85	Citizen who returned from Qom (Iran)
Pakistan	2020-02-26	87	Individuals who returned from Iran
Bhutan	2020-03-06	96	An American tourist who had a travel history in India
Bangladesh	2020-03-08	98	Two men who returned from Italy and a female relative

(Continued)

Country	First case date	Days since outbreak (1 December 2019)	First case description
Maldives	2020-03-08	98	Foreign employees at Kuredu Island Resort who were assumed to get the infection from an Italian tourist
Southeast Asia			
Thailand	2020-01-13	43	A Chinese female from Wuhan
Singapore	2020-01-23	53	A tourist from Wuhan
Vietnam	2020-01-23	53	A Chinese man flown from Wuhan to visit his son who was assumed to get the infection when they met
Malaysia	2020-01-25	55	A Chinese national who visited Malaysia
Cambodia	2020-01-27	57	A Chinese man from Wuhan
Philippines	2020-01-30	60	A Chinese woman from Wuhan who arrived via Hong Kong
Indonesia	2020-03-02	92	A dance instructor and her mother had held a dance class, which was attended by a Japanese, who later tested positive in Malaysia
Brunei	2020-03-09	99	A male who returned from Kuala Lumpur
Timor	2020-03-21	111	An individual who returned from abroad
Myanmar	2020-03-23	113	Myanmar citizens who returned from the US and the UK
Laos	2020-03-24	114	A man who had a travel history in Thailand
Western Asia			
The United Arab Emirates	2020-01-29	59	A Chinese female from Wuhan
Iran	2020-02-19	80	A merchant who returned from China
Bahrain	2020-02-21	82	A school bus driver from Iran via Dubai
Israel	2020-02-21	82	A female Israeli citizen who returned from Japan
Lebanon	2020-02-21	82	A female who returned from Iran
Kuwait	2020-02-24	85	A Kuwaiti man who returned from Iran
Oman	2020-02-24	85	Omani females who returned from Iran
Iraq	2020-02-24	85	An Iranian religious studies student
Georgia	2020-02-26	87	A man who returned from Iran
Qatar	2020-02-29	90	A Qatari male who returned from Iran
Azerbaijan	2020-03-01	91	A Russian national who had a travel history in Iran
Armenia	2020-03-01	91	An Armenian national who returned from Iran
Saudi Arabia	2020-03-02	92	A Saudi national who returned from Iran via Bahrain
Jordan	2020-03-03	93	A Jordanian who returned from Italy
Palestine	2020-03-05	95	A group of Greek tourists
Turkey	2020-03-11	101	A local who returned from Europe

(Continued)

Country	First case date	Days since outbreak (1 December 2019)	First case description
Syria	2020-03-22	112	An individual who had a travel history from abroad
Yemen	2020-04-10	131	A man in Hadhramaut
Central Europe			
Germany	2020-01-27	57	A German was infected by a Chinese colleague who was from China
Switzerland	2020-02-25	86	A man who had a travel history in Milan
Austria	2020-02-25	86	A male and a female who returned from Lombardy (Italy)
Czechia	2020-03-01	91	A man who returned from Udine; a US tourist who studied in Milan; and a man who returned from Auronzo di Cadore
Hungary	2020-03-04	94	Students from Iran studying in Hungary
Poland	2020-03-04	94	A man who returned from Germany
Liechtenstein	2020-03-04	94	A man who had contact with an infected person in Switzerland
Slovakia	2020-03-06	96	The patient had not been outside Slovakia but his son had a travel history in Venice (Italy)
East Europe			
Russia	2020-01-31	61	Two Chinese citizens in Tyumen (Siberia) and Chita (Russian Far East)
Estonia	2020-02-27	88	An Iranian citizen departed from Iran and flown from Turkey to Riga
Belarus	2020-02-28	89	An Iranian student
Lithuania	2020-02-29	90	A female who returned from Verona, Italy
Latvia	2020-03-02	92	A female who returned from Milan and Munich
Ukraine	2020-03-03	93	A man who had a travel history in Italy and Romania
North Europe			
Finland	2020-01-29	59	A Chinese tourist from Wuhan
Sweden	2020-01-31	61	A female who returned from Wuhan China
Norway	2020-02-26	87	An individual who returned from China
Denmark	2020-02-27	88	A man who returned from Lombardy (Italy)
Iceland	2020-02-28	89	An Icelandic male who returned from Northern Italy
Faeroe Islands	2020-03-04	94	A man who returned from Paris
Southern Europe			
Italy	2020-01-31	61	Two Chinese tourists

(Continued)

Country	First case date	Days since outbreak (1 December 2019)	First case description
Greece	2020-02-26	87	A female who returned from Northern Italy
San Marino	2020-02-27	88	The patient had no travel history
Vatican	2020-03-06	96	A priest who arrived from one of Italy's red zones
Malta	2020-03-07	97	An Italian national who arrived from the region of Trentino
Cyprus	2020-03-09	99	A man who returned from Italy and a heart surgeon who returned from England
Southeast Europe			
Croatia	2020-02-25	86	A man who stayed in Milan (Italy)
Romania	2020-02-26	87	The patient had a travel history in Italy
North Macedonia	2020-02-26	87	A female who had a travel history in Italy
Slovenia	2020-03-04	94	A tourist traveling from Morocco via Italy
Bosnia and Herzegovina	2020-03-05	95	A Bosnian who returned from Italy
Serbia	2020-03-06	96	A man who returned from Budapest
Bulgaria	2020-03-08	98	Two local Bulgarians who had no travel history in areas with known coronavirus cases
Moldova	2020-03-08	98	A female who returned from Italy
Albania	2020-03-09	99	A father and a son and the son had a travel history in Florence (Italy)
Kosovo	2020-03-14	104	A man from Vitina and an Italian woman who worked in Klina
Montenegro	2020-03-17	107	Citizens who returned from the US and Spain
Western Europe			
France	2020-01-24	54	A French citizen who returned from China
The United Kingdom	2020-01-31	61	Two Chinese nationals
Spain	2020-01-31	61	A German tourist in La Gomera, Canary Islands
Belgium	2020-02-04	65	Belgians who returned from Wuhan
The Netherlands	2020-02-27	88	A man who returned from the Lombardy region of Italy
Luxembourg	2020-02-29	90	A man who returned from Italy via Charleroi (Belgium)
Ireland	2020-02-29	90	A male student who returned from Northern Italy
Monaco	2020-02-29	90	

(*Continued*)

Country	First case date	Days since outbreak (1 December 2019)	First case description
Portugal	2020-03-02	92	A doctor who traveled to the north of Italy and a man working in Spain
Andorra	2020-03-02	92	An individual who returned from Milan (Italy)
Gibraltar	2020-03-04	94	A person who had a travel history in Northern Italy
Guernsey	2020-03-09	99	The patient had a travel history in Tenerife
Jersey	2020-03-10	100	An individual who returned from Italy
Isle of Man	2020-03-19	109	The patient had a travel history in Spain
Oceania			
Australia	2020-01-26	56	A man who returned from Wuhan (China)
New Zealand	2020-02-28	89	A female who returned from Iran
Fiji	2020-03-19	109	A Fijian citizen and a flight attendant of Fiji Airways who returned from San Francisco
Papua New Guinea	2020-03-20	110	A man who had a travel history in Spain
Solomon Islands	2020-10-03	307	A student repatriated from the Philippines
Marshall Islands	2020-10-28	332	Members of the US Army Garrison
Vanuatu	2020-11-10	345	A man who had a travel history in the US, Sydney, and Auckland
Samoa	2020-11-18	353	A sailor who returned from Auckland (New Zealand)
Micronesia (country)	2021-01-11	407	A crew member on a government ship "Chief Mailo" which had been in the Philippines

Source: Compiled by authors from various online sources.

Appendix-II: Country-wise early response to COVID-19

Country	First case	First death		Vaccination programs launch	
	Date	Date	Days since first case	Date	Days since outbreak (1 December 2019)
Caribbean					
Dominican Republic	2020-03-01	2020-03-17	16	2021-02-16	443
Jamaica	2020-03-11	2020-03-19	8	2021-03-10	465
Saint Vincent and the Grenadines	2020-03-11	2021-01-15	310	NA	
Cayman Islands	2020-03-12	2020-03-14	2	2021-01-08	404
Trinidad and Tobago	2020-03-12	2020-03-25	13	2021-02-17	444
Cuba	2020-03-12	2020-03-18	6		
Antigua and Barbuda	2020-03-13	2020-04-04	22	2021-02-17	444
Saint Lucia	2020-03-13	2020-11-10	242	2021-02-17	444
Bahamas	2020-03-16	2020-04-01	16	2021-03-14	469
Barbados	2020-03-17	2020-04-05	19	2021-02-15	442
Montserrat	2020-03-18	2020-04-24	37	2021-02-08	435
Haiti	2020-03-20	2020-04-05	16	2020-12-24	389
Grenada	2020-03-22	2021-01-03	287	2021-02-13	440
Dominica	2020-03-22			2021-02-24	451
Turks and Caicos Islands	2020-03-23	2020-04-05	13	2021-01-11	407
Anguilla	2020-03-24	2020-04-23	30	2021-02-05	432
Saint Kitts and Nevis	2020-03-24			2021-02-25	452
Central America					
Costa Rica	2020-03-06	2020-03-19	13	2020-12-24	389
Panama	2020-03-10	2020-03-11	1	2021-01-20	416
Honduras	2020-03-11	2020-03-26	15	2021-02-27	454
Guatemala	2020-03-14	2020-03-16	2	2021-02-27	454
Nicaragua	2020-03-19	2020-03-27	8	2021-04-05	491
El Salvador	2020-03-19	2020-03-31	12	2021-02-17	444

(Continued)

Country	First case	First death		Vaccination programs launch	
	Date	Date	Days since first case	Date	Days since outbreak (1 December 2019)
Belize	2020-03-23	2020-04-04	12	2021-03-02	457
North America					
The United States	2020-01-21	2020-02-06	16	2020-12-14	379
Canada	2020-01-26	2020-03-09	43	2020-12-14	379
Mexico	2020-02-28	2020-03-19	20	2020-12-24	389
Greenland	2020-03-16			2021-01-04	400
Bermuda	2020-03-18	2020-04-06	19	2021-01-11	407
South America					
Brazil	2020-02-26	2020-03-17	20	2021-01-17	413
Ecuador	2020-03-01	2020-03-14	13	2021-01-22	418
Chile	2020-03-03	2020-03-22	19	2020-12-24	389
Argentina	2020-03-03	2020-03-08	5	2020-12-29	394
Peru	2020-03-06	2020-03-20	14	2021-02-09	436
Colombia	2020-03-06	2020-03-22	16	2021-02-17	444
Paraguay	2020-03-08	2020-03-21	13	2021-02-22	449
Bolivia	2020-03-11	2020-03-29	18	2021-01-29	425
Guyana	2020-03-12	2020-03-12	0	2021-02-11	438
Suriname	2020-03-13	2020-04-03	21	2021-02-23	450
Uruguay	2020-03-13	2020-03-28	15	2021-03-01	456
Venezuela	2020-03-14	2020-03-27	13	2021-02-18	445
Falkland Islands	2020-04-03			2021-02-08	435
Central Africa					
Cameroon	2020-03-06	2020-03-25	19	2021-04-12	498
Democratic Republic of Congo	2020-03-11	2020-03-21	10	2021-04-19	505
Gabon	2020-03-12	2020-03-20	8	2021-03-24	479
Equatorial Guinea	2020-03-15	2020-04-20	36	2021-02-15	442
Central African Republic	2020-03-15	2020-05-23	69		
Congo	2020-03-15	2020-03-31	16		
Chad	2020-03-19	2020-04-28	40		
Angola	2020-03-20	2020-03-29	9	2021-03-09	464
Sao Tome and Principe	2020-04-06	2020-04-30	24	NA	
East Africa					
Kenya	2020-03-13	2020-03-26	13	2021-03-05	460
Sudan	2020-03-13	2020-03-12	-1	2021-03-11	466
Ethiopia	2020-03-13	2020-04-05	23	2021-03-13	468
Seychelles	2020-03-14	2021-01-03	295	2021-01-10	406
Rwanda	2020-03-14	2020-05-31	78	2021-03-05	460
Somalia	2020-03-16	2020-04-08	23	2021-03-16	471
Tanzania	2020-03-16	2020-03-31	15		

(*Continued*)

Country	First case	First death		Vaccination programs launch	
	Date	Date	Days since first case	Date	Days since outbreak (1 December 2019)
Mauritius	2020-03-18	2020-03-21	3	2021-01-26	422
Djibouti	2020-03-18	2020-04-10	23	2021-03-15	470
Zambia	2020-03-18	2020-04-02	15	2021-04-14	500
Zimbabwe	2020-03-20	2020-03-23	3	2021-02-22	449
Madagascar	2020-03-20	2020-05-17	58		
Eritrea	2020-03-21	2020-12-22	276		
Mozambique	2020-03-22	2020-05-25	64	2021-03-08	463
Uganda	2020-03-22	2020-07-23	123	2021-03-10	465
Burundi	2020-03-31	2020-04-13	13		
Malawi	2020-04-02	2020-04-07	5	2021-03-11	466
South Sudan	2020-04-05	2020-05-14	39	2021-04-06	492
Comoros	2020-04-30	2020-05-04	4	2021-04-10	496
North Africa					
Egypt	2020-02-14	2020-03-08	23	2021-01-24	420
Algeria	2020-02-25	2020-03-12	16	2021-01-30	426
Morocco	2020-03-02	2020-03-10	8	2021-01-28	424
Tunisia	2020-03-02	2020-03-19	17	2021-03-13	468
Libya	2020-03-24	2020-04-02	9	2021-04-10	496
Southern Africa					
South Africa	2020-03-05	2020-03-27	22	2021-02-18	445
Namibia	2020-03-14	2020-07-10	118	2021-03-19	474
Eswatini	2020-03-14	2020-04-16	33	2021-03-24	479
Botswana	2020-03-30	2020-03-31	1	2021-03-26	481
Lesotho	2020-05-13	2020-07-09	57	2021-03-10	465
West Africa					
Nigeria	2020-02-28	2020-03-23	24	2021-03-05	460
Senegal	2020-03-02	2020-03-31	29	2021-02-23	450
Togo	2020-03-06	2020-03-27	21	2021-03-10	465
Burkina Faso	2020-03-10	2020-03-18	8		
Cote d'Ivoire	2020-03-11	2020-03-29	18	2021-03-01	456
Ghana	2020-03-12	2020-03-21	9	2021-03-01	456
Guinea	2020-03-13	2020-04-15	33	2021-01-15	411
Mauritania	2020-03-14	2020-03-30	16	2021-03-26	481
Benin	2020-03-16	2020-04-06	21	2021-03-29	484
Liberia	2020-03-16	2020-04-04	19	2021-04-01	487
Gambia	2020-03-17	2020-03-23	6	2021-03-10	465
Cape Verde	2020-03-20	2020-03-24	4	2021-03-18	473
Niger	2020-03-20	2020-03-25	5	2021-03-29	484
Mali	2020-03-25	2020-03-29	4	2021-03-31	486
Guinea-Bissau	2020-03-25	2020-04-26	32	2021-04-03	489
Sierra Leone	2020-03-31	2020-04-23	23	2021-03-15	470
Central Asia					
Kazakhstan	2020-03-13	2020-03-26	13	2021-02-01	428

(*Continued*)

Country	First case	First death		Vaccination programs launch	
	Date	Date	Days since first case	Date	Days since outbreak (1 December 2019)
Uzbekistan	2020-03-15	2020-03-27	12	2021-04-01	487
Kyrgyzstan	2020-03-18	2020-04-03	16	2021-03-29	484
Tajikistan	2020-04-30	2020-05-02	2	2021-03-23	478
East Asia					
China	2019-12-01	2020-01-09	39	2020-12-15	380
Japan	2020-01-15	2020-02-13	29	2021-02-17	444
South Korea	2020-01-20	2020-02-20	31	2021-02-26	453
Taiwan	2020-01-21	2020-02-16	26	2021-03-22	477
Mongolia	2020-03-10	2020-12-30	295	2021-02-23	450
South Asia					
Nepal	2020-01-23	2020-05-14	112	2021-01-27	423
Sri Lanka	2020-01-27	2020-03-28	61	2021-01-29	425
India	2020-01-30	2020-03-12	42	2021-01-16	412
Afghanistan	2020-02-24	2020-03-22	27	2021-02-28	455
Pakistan	2020-02-26	2020-03-18	21	2021-02-02	429
Bhutan	2020-03-06	2021-01-08	308	2021-03-27	482
Bangladesh	2020-03-08	2020-03-18	10	2021-01-27	423
Maldives	2020-03-08	2020-04-30	53	2021-02-02	429
Southeast Asia					
Thailand	2020-01-13	2020-03-01	48	2021-02-28	455
Singapore	2020-01-23	2020-03-21	58	2020-12-30	395
Vietnam	2020-01-23	2020-07-31	190	2021-03-08	463
Malaysia	2020-01-25	2020-03-17	52	2021-02-24	451
Cambodia	2020-01-27	2021-03-11	409	2021-02-10	437
Philippines	2020-01-30	2020-02-01	2	2021-03-01	456
Indonesia	2020-03-02	2020-03-11	9	2021-01-13	409
Brunei	2020-03-09	2020-03-27	18	2021-04-01	487
Timor	2020-03-21	2021-04-06	381	2021-04-07	493
Myanmar	2020-03-23	2020-03-31	8	2021-01-27	423
Laos	2020-03-24			NA	472
Western Asia					
The United Arab Emirates	2020-01-29	2020-03-20	51	2020-12-14	379
Iran	2020-02-19	2020-02-19	0	2021-02-09	436
Bahrain	2020-02-21	2020-03-16	24	2020-12-17	382
Israel	2020-02-21	2020-03-20	28	2020-12-19	384
Lebanon	2020-02-21	2020-03-10	18	2021-02-14	441
Kuwait	2020-02-24	2020-04-04	40	2020-12-24	389
Oman	2020-02-24	2020-03-31	36	2020-12-27	392
Iraq	2020-02-24	2020-03-04	9	2021-03-02	457
Georgia	2020-02-26	2020-03-12	15	2021-03-18	473
Qatar	2020-02-29	2020-03-28	28	2020-12-23	388
Azerbaijan	2020-03-01	2020-03-13	12	2021-02-06	433

(*Continued*)

Country	First case	First death		Vaccination programs launch	
	Date	Date	Days since first case	Date	Days since outbreak (1 December 2019)
Armenia	2020-03-01	2020-03-26	25	2021-04-13	499
Saudi Arabia	2020-03-02	2020-03-24	22	2020-12-17	382
Jordan	2020-03-03	2020-03-27	24	2021-01-13	409
Palestine	2020-03-05	2020-03-26	21	2021-02-22	449
Turkey	2020-03-11	2020-03-15	4	2021-01-13	409
Syria	2020-03-22	2020-03-29	7	not confirm	
Yemen	2020-04-10	2020-04-30	20	2021-04-20	506
Central Europe					
Germany	2020-01-27	2020-03-09	42	2020-12-27	392
Switzerland	2020-02-25	2020-03-05	9	2020-12-23	388
Austria	2020-02-25	2020-03-12	16	2020-12-27	392
Czechia	2020-03-01	2020-03-22	21	2020-12-27	392
Hungary	2020-03-04	2020-03-15	11	2020-12-26	391
Poland	2020-03-04	2020-03-12	8	2020-12-26	391
Liechtenstein	2020-03-04	2020-04-04	31	2021-01-18	414
Slovakia	2020-03-06	2020-03-30	24	2020-12-26	391
Eastern Europe					
Russia	2020-01-31	2020-03-19	48	2020-12-05	370
Estonia	2020-02-27	2020-03-25	27	2020-12-28	393
Belarus	2020-02-28	2020-03-31	32	2020-12-29	394
Lithuania	2020-02-29	2020-03-20	20	2020-12-27	392
Latvia	2020-03-02	2020-04-03	32	2020-12-28	393
Ukraine	2020-03-03	2020-03-13	10	2021-02-24	451
Northern Europe					
Finland	2020-01-29	2020-03-21	52	2020-12-27	392
Sweden	2020-01-31	2020-03-11	40	2020-12-27	392
Norway	2020-02-26	2020-03-12	15	2020-12-27	392
Denmark	2020-02-27	2020-03-14	16	2020-12-27	392
Iceland	2020-02-28	2020-03-24	25	2020-12-30	395
Faeroe Islands	2020-03-04	2021-01-05	307	2020-12-30	395
Southern Europe					
Italy	2020-01-31	2020-02-21	21	2020-12-31	396
Greece	2020-02-26	2020-03-11	14	2020-12-28	393
San Marino	2020-02-27	2020-03-01	3	2021-02-25	452
Vatican	2020-03-06			2021-01-13	409
Malta	2020-03-07	2020-04-08	32	2020-12-27	392
Cyprus	2020-03-09	2020-03-22	13	2020-12-27	392
Southeast Europe					
Croatia	2020-02-25	2020-03-19	23	2020-12-27	392
Romania	2020-02-26	2020-03-22	25	2020-12-27	392
North Macedonia	2020-02-26	2020-03-22	25	2021-02-17	444
Slovenia	2020-03-04	2020-03-14	10	2020-12-27	392
Bosnia and Herzegovina	2020-03-05	2020-03-21	16	2021-02-12	439

(Continued)

Country	First case	First death		Vaccination programs launch	
	Date	Date	Days since first case	Date	Days since outbreak (1 December 2019)
Serbia	2020-03-06	2020-03-20	14	2020-12-24	389
Bulgaria	2020-03-08	2020-03-11	3	2020-12-27	392
Moldova	2020-03-08	2020-03-18	10	2021-03-02	457
Albania	2020-03-09	2020-03-11	2	2021-01-12	408
Kosovo	2020-03-14	2020-03-23	9	2021-03-29	484
Montenegro	2020-03-17	2020-03-23	6	2021-02-21	448
Western Europe					
France	2020-01-24	2020-02-15	22	2020-12-27	392
The United Kingdom	2020-01-31	2020-03-05	34	2020-12-08	373
Spain	2020-01-31	2020-02-13	13	2020-12-27	392
Belgium	2020-02-04	2020-03-11	36	2020-12-28	393
The Netherlands	2020-02-27	2020-03-06	8	2021-01-06	402
Luxembourg	2020-02-29	2020-03-14	14	2020-12-28	393
Ireland	2020-02-29	2020-03-11	11	2020-12-29	394
Monaco	2020-02-29	2020-03-29	29	2021-01-19	415
Portugal	2020-03-02	2020-03-16	14	2020-12-27	392
Andorra	2020-03-02	2020-03-22	20	2021-01-26	422
Gibraltar	2020-03-04	2020-11-11	252	2021-01-10	406
Guernsey	2020-03-09	2020-03-30	21	2020-12-17	382
Jersey	2020-03-10	2020-03-15	5	2020-12-13	378
Isle of Man	2020-03-19	2020-04-01	13	2021-01-04	400
Oceania					
Australia	2020-01-26	2020-03-01	35	2021-02-22	449
New Zealand	2020-02-28	2020-03-29	30	2021-02-19	446
Fiji	2020-03-19	2020-07-31	134	2021-03-10	465
Papua New Guinea	2020-03-20	2020-07-27	129	2021-03-30	485
Solomon Islands	2020-10-03			2021-03-24	479
Marshall Islands	2020-10-28			2020-12-29	394
Vanuatu	2020-11-10				
Samoa	2020-11-18			NA	
Micronesia (country)	2021-01-11			2020-12-31	396

Source: Compiled by authors from various online sources. NA = Not available.

Mini-case I: Samsung response to COVID-19

Samsung Electronics is a South Korean multinational company and one of the world's largest manufacturers and sellers of mobile phones (Samsung, 2023). During the COVID-19 outbreak, it was inevitable that as part of the devastating impact on almost every sector of the global economy, the supply chain disruption, retail store closures, and prolonged economic downturn, also damaged the consumer electronics business. In this mini-case, we use the example of Samsung Electronics to see how its mobile phone business adapted to the rapidly changing business environment to minimize the negative impact of COVID-19 on its operations.

Supply during pandemic

With rapid growth in the global economy in the last few decades, supply chain systems have become more and more complex and interconnected (Panwar et al., 2022). Interestingly, the World Economic Forum's Supply Chain and Transport Risk Survey (WEF, 2012) predicted that a global pandemic could be one of the key triggers to cause global supply chain disruptions. In addition, the tsunami of Sumatra in 2004 and Fukushima in 2011 were wake-up calls for many multinationals to learn lessons about the weaknesses in their supply chains. However, it appears that most companies were caught unaware of and unprepared for COVID-19 and unsurprisingly, it proved to be a very painful lesson for those companies that were not prepared enough for a pervasive supply chain disruption (Moosavi et al., 2022).

China has become well-known as the world's factory and production powerhouse for the manufacture of many products, such as electronics, consumer goods, and medical supplies, in the past few decades. However, Samsung Electronics realized the risks of relying on China as a single source for its mobile phone components and as the only manufacturing center for its products. Therefore, Samsung Electronics has established a vast manufacturing network over the years in order to fulfill its huge production demand. For example, its factories for smartphones are located in several countries, including Brazil, India, Indonesia, South Korea, and Vietnam, which incidentally are also the largest markets for its mobile phones. In fact, all its factories in China were actually closed by the end of 2019. Moreover, Samsung Electronics had to temporarily close its factories in other countries during the outbreak due to the requests from the governments in those countries. However, since the shutdowns of factories in various locations were just temporary and in different time periods, the production process could be shifted from one location to another, which resulted only in a slowdown in production and not a complete shutdown. This was a testament to the foresight and advance planning by Samsung Electronics to diversify its manufacturing.

Sales during pandemic

Due to the closure of the retail stores, Samsung Electronics signed partnership agreements with other companies, including mobile phone retailers and even Benow (a payment and EMI technology firm) to create an e-commerce platform, so that the retail business can still continue to sell and deliver the products to consumers (Mukherjee, 2020). In order to maintain the relationship and keep the loyal support of the consumers, Samsung Electronics launched additional services for its consumers. For example, to appreciate the continued services provided by the healthcare professionals, Samsung Electronics USA provided a "Free Repairs for the Frontline" program to offer free smartphone repair service for them until 30 June 2020 (Samsung, 2020). In addition, the first responders and healthcare professionals could enjoy new special discounts for online purchases (Mihai, 2020). Samsung Electronics plans to have its "Galaxy Sanitizing Service" for Samsung smartphones, watches, and buds by using UV-C light for free for Samsung consumers at its service centers (Eadicicco, 2020). This new service helped fight the spread of virus during the COVID-19 outbreak but is also relevant to keep mobile devices clean even in the post-pandemic era.

Innovation during pandemic

Samsung Galaxy Watch Active 2 is a smartwatch launched by Samsung Electronics (Samsung, 2019). The watch was designed to be a lifestyle and health partner for the customers. One of the selling points of the watch is to provide information on health and wellness such as the skin temperature, heart rates and rhythm, blood pressure, and other physiological conditions of the customers. Samsung Electronics South Africa collaborated with 1Life and LifeQ to launch a "Covid-19 Screening App" using the Samsung Galaxy Watch Active 2 Device. The aim of the App was to help contain the spread of the virus. The App could enable the users to take proactive precautionary measures in the event of a likely outbreak of COVID-19 by notifying the users if they have the possible symptoms of the virus. The App combined the data collection functions of Samsung Galaxy Watch Active 2 to collect the physiological indicators of the users and the analysis functions of LifeQ's software to evaluate the changes in the health biometrics of the users. In this way, the App can serve a detection purpose to identify the existence of COVID-19 infections sometime before the users show COVID-19 symptoms so as to alert the users about the changes in their biometrics.

References

Eadicicco, L. (2020). Samsung is offering to clean your smartphone for free as the coronavirus continues to spread. *Business Insider*, (13 March 2020). https://www. businessinsider.com/samsung-sanitizing-service-launch-clean-phone-coronavirus-2020-3

Mihai, M. (2020). Samsung USA offers free device repairs to COVID-19 first responders, (22 April 2020). https://www.sammobile.com/news/samsung-usa-free-device-repairs-covid-19-first-responders/.

Moosavi, J., Fathollahi-Fard, A. M., & Dulebenets, M. A. (2022). Supply chain disruption during the COVID-19 pandemic: Recognizing potential disruption management strategies. *International Journal of Disaster Risk Reduction, 75*, 102983.

Mukherjee, W. (2020). Covid-19 fear: Electronics brands Samsung, Apple let offline stores sell online. *The Economic Times*, India, 18 April 2020.

Panwar, R., Pinkse, J., & De Marchi, V. (2022). The future of global supply chains in a post-COVID-19 world. *California Management Review, 64*(2), 5–23.

Samsung. (2019). Samsung Galaxy Watch Active 2. https://www.samsung. com/au/business/watches/galaxy-watch-active/galaxy-watch-active2-r820-sm-r820nzkaxsa/

Samsung. (2020). Caring for those who care for us. Samsung USA. https://news. samsung. com/us/samsung-free-repairs-frontline-initiative-covid19

Samsung. (2023). Samsung Global. https://www.samsung.com/about-us/company-info/

WEF. (2012). New models for addressing supply chain and transport risk. *World Economic Forum: Industry Agenda.*

Mini-case II: Digital payments revolution in India

Background

India started its journey towards a significant transformation in the digital payments landscape in the last decade and witnessed a rapid surge in digital payments, driven by several factors, including government initiatives, technological advancements, and changing consumer behaviors (Roy & Sahoo, 2016). The demonetization move in 2016, where high-denomination currency notes were invalidated, acted as a catalyst for the adoption of digital payment methods (Sivathanu, 2019). However, it experienced a rapid acceleration in this process during COVID-19 due to a number of factors (Chaudhari & Kumar, 2021). This mini-case examines the key players, milestones, challenges, and future outlook for the growth of digital payments systems in India and draws some useful lessons for managers.

Key players

Unified Payments Interface (UPI): UPI is a real-time payment system that allows users to link multiple bank accounts to a single mobile application, which has simplified peer-to-peer transactions and made digital payments more accessible (Sujith & Julie, 2017).

Mobile wallets: Companies like Paytm, Google Pay, PhonePe, and others have gained prominence as popular mobile wallet providers. These wallets offer a range of services, including bill payments, mobile recharges, and even offline transactions at various merchants.

Government initiatives: The Indian government has been actively promoting digital payments through initiatives like Digital India and Jan Dhan Yojana. Direct Benefit Transfer (DBT) programs have also contributed to increased digital transactions.

Case highlights

Demonetization impact: The demonetization move in 2016 led to a surge in digital payments as people looked for alternative ways to transact in the absence of physical currency. This prompted many to adopt mobile wallets and digital payment apps.

UPI growth: The launch of UPI by the National Payments Corporation of India (NPCI) has witnessed exponential growth. UPI transactions have become a preferred choice for users due to their simplicity and seamless inter-bank transfers.

Mobile wallet adoption: Mobile wallet providers like Paytm experienced rapid adoption. Paytm, in particular, expanded its services beyond payments, including offering digital financial services like insurance and investment products.

Rise of contactless payments: Contactless payments, facilitated by Near Field Communication (NFC) technology, gained traction. This was especially relevant during the COVID-19 pandemic when contactless transactions were encouraged for safety reasons.

Government subsidies and benefits: The government's push for direct transfers of subsidies and benefits to citizens' bank accounts encouraged the use of digital payment platforms. This streamlined the distribution process and reduced leakages.

Digital lending and finance: The digital payments ecosystem paved the way for digital lending and other financial services. Many fintech companies emerged to provide instant loans and other financial products based on individuals' digital transaction histories.

Challenges and future outlook

Security concerns: The growth of digital payments has raised concerns about cybersecurity and fraud. It emphasizes the need for robust security measures to protect users' financial data.

Digital literacy: Despite significant progress, there is a need for continued efforts in enhancing digital literacy, especially in rural areas, to ensure more widespread adoption of digital payment methods.

Regulatory landscape: The regulatory environment continues to evolve to address the challenges and opportunities in the digital payments space. Regulations need to strike a balance between fostering innovation and ensuring consumer protection.

Technology integration: Integration of emerging technologies like blockchain and artificial intelligence in digital payment systems is expected to shape the future of the industry, offering more efficient and secure transactions.

To conclude, the digital payments landscape in India has undergone a transformative journey, driven by technological advancements, government initiatives, and changing consumer preferences. The continued growth of digital payments is expected to contribute to a more inclusive and efficient financial ecosystem in the country.

References

Chaudhari, C., & Kumar, A. (2021). Study of impact of the covid-19 outbreak on digital payment in India. *Vidyabharati International Interdisciplinary Research Journal, 12*(02), 99–102.

Roy, D., & Sahoo, A. (2016). Payment systems in India: Opportunities and challenges. *Journal of Internet Banking and Commerce, 21*(2), 1–48.

Sivathanu, B. (2019). Adoption of digital payment systems in the era of demonetization in India: An empirical study. *Journal of Science and Technology Policy Management, 10*(1), 143–171.

Sujith T. S., & Julie C. D. (2017). Opportunities and challenges e-payment system in India. *International Journal of Scientific Research and Management (IJSRM), 5*(09), 6935–6943.

Mini-case III: JobKeeper Payment program in Australia

Background

The JobKeeper Payment was introduced by the Australian government in March 2020 as part of its economic response to the impact of the COVID-19 pandemic on businesses and employment (Borland & Hunt, 2023). The program aimed to provide financial assistance to eligible businesses to help them retain employees during a period of economic uncertainty (Walkowiak, 2021). JobKeeper Payment in Australia was a significant economic stimulus measure implemented in response to the COVID-19 pandemic (Australian Treasury, 2023). This mini-case provides an overview of the JobKeeper Payment program, its key features, challenges, outcomes, and future implications.

Key features

Employer eligibility: The JobKeeper Payment was available to eligible employers significantly affected by the economic impact of COVID-19. This included businesses experiencing a specified decline in their turnover.

Employee eligibility: Eligible employees included full-time and part-time workers, as well as casual employees who had been with their employer for at least 12 months. Sole traders and certain other self-employed individuals were also eligible.

Payment amounts: The JobKeeper Payment provided a flat-rate wage subsidy per eligible employee. Initially set at $1,500 per fortnight, the payment aimed to help employers continue paying their staff during the economic downturn.

Payment period: The program was initially intended to run for a specified period, with payments made for eligible employees for up to six months. However, the government extended the program multiple times in response to the ongoing impact of the pandemic.

Application process: Employers needed to apply for the JobKeeper Payment and demonstrate their eligibility based on the specified decline in turnover. The Australian Taxation Office (ATO) managed the application and payment processes.

Flexibility for employers: The program allowed employers to keep employees on the payroll, even if they had reduced working hours or were stood down. This flexibility aimed to prevent widespread job losses during the economic downturn.

Case highlights

Economic support: The JobKeeper Payment played a crucial role in providing economic support to businesses and employees affected by the pandemic. It helped stabilize the labor market during a period of uncertainty and reduced the financial burden on employers.

Business continuity: Many businesses were able to maintain their operations and keep employees on the payroll with the help of the JobKeeper Payment. This contributed to business continuity and preserved the employer-employee relationship.

Government adaptation: The Australian government demonstrated flexibility by extending the program in response to the evolving nature of the pandemic. The extensions provided ongoing support to businesses facing prolonged challenges.

Challenges and controversies: The program faced challenges and controversies, including issues related to eligibility criteria, concerns about potential misuse, and debates about the effectiveness of the program in certain sectors.

Outcomes and future implications

Impact on unemployment: The JobKeeper Payment contributed to preventing a more significant increase in unemployment rates during the initial phases of the pandemic. It provided a safety net for businesses to retain employees.

Economic recovery: The program was part of the broader economic recovery strategy in Australia. As the country navigated through different phases of the pandemic, ongoing economic support measures were introduced to facilitate recovery.

Policy evaluation: The JobKeeper Payment program underwent evaluations to assess its effectiveness and identify areas for improvement. Lessons learned from the implementation of the program could inform future policy responses to economic crises.

Transition plans: As economic conditions improved, there were discussions about transitioning away from direct wage subsidies and focusing on other forms of economic stimulus to support recovery.

To conclude, the JobKeeper Payment program in Australia played a crucial role in providing financial assistance to businesses and employees impacted by the COVID-19 pandemic. It was designed to support economic stability, business continuity, and job retention during a period of unprecedented challenges. For the most current and detailed information, it is advisable to refer to the latest reports and updates from official government sources or relevant authorities in Australia.

References

Australian Treasury. (2023). Independent evaluation of the JobKeeper Payment. *Consultation Paper* (16 June 2023). https://treasury.gov.au/sites/default/files/2023-06/c2023-407908.pdf

Borland, J., & Hunt, J. (2023). JobKeeper: An initial assessment. *Australian Economic Review*, *56*(1), 109–123.

Walkowiak, E. (2021). JobKeeper: The Australian short-time work program. *Australian Journal of Public Administration*, *80*(4), 1046–1053.

Mini-case IV: COVID-19 vaccine diplomacy

The Indian experience

Background

One of the most interesting sideshows to the COVID-19 pandemic was the concept of "vaccine diplomacy" (Hotez & Narayan, 2021), with many nations using their strengths in vaccine manufacturing and distribution as a means to advance their geopolitical interests (Sparke & Levy, 2022; Su et al., 2021). For example, India has been a key player in the global fight against the COVID-19 pandemic providing 60% of the global vaccine supply (Sharun & Dhama, 2021) and emerged as a global vaccine hub with its capacity to manufacture more than three billion COVID-19 vaccines doses per annum (Bharti & Bharti, 2021; Sharma & Varshney, 2021). As part of its vaccine diplomacy efforts, India not only shared its homegrown vaccines with low-income countries (Singh et al., 2023) but also supplied its vaccines to more developed countries like Australia, the Netherlands, and the UK, with total exports of more than 300 million doses (Sharun & Dhama, 2021). Interestingly, China also tried vaccine diplomacy to repair the damage to its image during the pandemic and to strengthen its global position as a growing economic and geopolitical power, albeit with mixed success (Apolinário Júnior et al., 2022; Suzuki & Yang, 2023). This mini-case describes India's successful development of its own COVID-19 vaccines and attempts to establish itself as a leader in global vaccine market.

India's emergence as a leading vaccine manufacturer

Development and approval: India played a significant role in COVID-19 vaccine development. Two vaccines developed in India gained widespread attention: Covishield (the Oxford-AstraZeneca vaccine manufactured by the Serum Institute of India) and Covaxin (developed by Bharat Biotech in collaboration with the Indian Council of Medical Research). These vaccines went through rigorous testing and received approval for emergency use.

Production capacity: India's pharmaceutical industry, known for its robust manufacturing capabilities, played a crucial role in producing large quantities of COVID-19 vaccines. The Serum Institute of India, in particular, became a major global supplier of vaccines.

Global distribution: India embarked on a mission called "Vaccine Maitri", meaning Vaccine Friendship, to supply COVID-19 vaccines to various countries. This initiative aimed to assist nations, particularly in the developing world, in their vaccination efforts.

Domestic vaccination drive: India launched one of the world's largest vaccination drives to inoculate its own population. The campaign involved setting up vaccination centers across the country and prioritizing high-risk groups, including healthcare workers and the elderly.

Digital platform: India utilized a digital platform called CoWIN (COVID Vaccine Intelligence Network) to manage and track the vaccination process. This platform allowed individuals to register for vaccination, schedule appointments, and receive digital certificates.

Public-private collaboration: The success of India's COVID-19 vaccination efforts was facilitated by strong collaborations between the government and private sector entities. Public and private healthcare facilities were actively involved in the vaccination drive.

Key highlights

Speedy rollout: India's vaccination campaign demonstrated a rapid and efficient rollout, with millions of doses administered within a short period. The country achieved significant milestones in terms of the number of doses administered daily.

Global impact: India's "Vaccine Maitri" initiative earned international acclaim for its efforts in supplying vaccines to other countries. This global outreach was seen as a testament to India's commitment to global public health.

Affordability and accessibility: India's vaccine production contributed to global efforts to ensure vaccine affordability and accessibility, especially for developing nations. The Serum Institute's commitment to producing large volumes at a low cost played a crucial role in this.

Adaptability and innovation: India showcased adaptability and innovation in managing its vaccination drive, including the use of technology for registration and tracking, as well as the deployment of mobile vaccination units to reach remote areas.

Challenges and lessons learned

Logistical challenges: Despite successes, there were logistical challenges in ensuring the smooth distribution of vaccines to all parts of the country, especially in remote areas. Addressing these challenges required ongoing efforts.

Vaccine hesitancy: Vaccine hesitancy was observed in some segments of the population. Public awareness campaigns were implemented to address misinformation and encourage vaccine acceptance.

Global supply chain issues: The global nature of vaccine distribution faced challenges related to supply chain disruptions. Ensuring a stable supply of vaccine components and raw materials was crucial.

Equitable distribution: The importance of equitable distribution both within the country and globally emerged as a critical consideration. Efforts were made to ensure that vulnerable populations and underserved communities were not left behind.

Outcomes and future implications

Global health diplomacy: India's vaccine success elevated its status in global health diplomacy. The country emerged as a key contributor to the global fight against the pandemic, showcasing its capabilities in vaccine production and distribution.

Strengthening healthcare infrastructure: The vaccination campaign highlighted the need for ongoing investments in healthcare infrastructure, including vaccination centers, cold storage facilities, and digital platforms for efficient management.

Role of innovation and collaboration: The success of India's COVID-19 vaccine efforts underscored the importance of innovation, collaboration between public and private sectors, and global cooperation in addressing health crises.

Preparedness for future pandemics: The experiences gained from the COVID-19 vaccination drive positioned India to be better prepared for future pandemics. The lessons learned could help the Indian government and vaccine manufacturing companies develop strategies for vaccine development, distribution, and public health management.

To conclude, India's success in developing, producing, and distributing COVID-19 vaccines marks a major milestone in the global response to the pandemic. The country's efforts not only protected its own population but also contributed to the broader global effort to achieve widespread vaccination and combat the impact of COVID-19. For the most current and detailed information, it is advisable to refer to the latest reports and updates from official sources.

References

Apolinário Júnior, L., Rinaldi, A. L., & Lima, R. D. C. (2022). Chinese and Indian COVID-19 vaccine diplomacy during the health emergency crisis. *Revista Brasileira De Política Internacional*, 65(1), e014.

Bharti, S. S., & Bharti, S. S. (2021). India's vaccine diplomacy: Role in new order and challenges. *Torun International Studies*, 1(14), 93–104.

Hotez, P. J., & Narayan, K. V. (2021). Restoring vaccine diplomacy. *Journal of the American Medical Association*, 325(23), 2337–2338.

Sharma, J., & Varshney, S. K. (2021). India's vaccine diplomacy aids global access to COVID-19 jabs.

Sharun, K., & Dhama, K. (2021). COVID-19 vaccine diplomacy and equitable access to vaccines amid ongoing pandemic. *Archives of Medical Research*, *52*(7), 761–763.

Singh, B., Singh, S., Singh, B., & Chattu, V. K. (2023). India's neighbourhood vaccine diplomacy during COVID-19 pandemic: Humanitarian and geopolitical perspectives. *Journal of Asian and African Studies*, *58*(6), 1021–1037.

Sparke, M., & Levy, O. (2022). Competing responses to global inequalities in access to COVID vaccines: Vaccine diplomacy and vaccine charity versus vaccine liberty. *Clinical Infectious Diseases*, *75*(S1), S86–S92.

Su, Z., McDonnell, D., Li, X., Bennett, B., Šegalo, S., Abbas, J., Cheshmehzangi, A., & Xiang, Y. T. (2021). COVID-19 vaccine donations—Vaccine empathy or vaccine diplomacy? A narrative literature review. *Vaccines*, *9*(9), 1024.

Suzuki, M., & Yang, S. (2023). Political economy of vaccine diplomacy: Explaining varying strategies of China, India, and Russia's COVID-19 vaccine diplomacy. *Review of International Political Economy*, *30*(3), 865–890.

Index

Note: Page numbers in italics denote figures. Page numbers of boldface denote tables.

Access to COVID-19 Tools (ACT) Accelerator 56
adaptability 1–2, 17, 32, 41, 54, 69, 89, 92–93, 102–103, 105–106, 112, 115, 119, 121–123, 129, 138, 142, 188
agility 89, 105–106, 121, 127
antibody test 43
antigen test 43, *44*
anxiety *6*, 11, 26–27, *28*, 29–31, 53, 65–66, 109
artificial intelligence (AI) 17, 24, 41–42, 52, 91, 112, 182
automation 21, 91, 93–94, 129, 131

blanket lockdown 65
blended learning 26
blockchain 41, 90, 93, 111, 182
booster 13, 62, 65, 67–69
border closure 2, 23, 45–46, 49, 71
border control 46, 64
burnout 6, 30, 60, 66, 109
business closure 7, 20, 23, 29, 32, 40, 51, 53, 66
business continuity management system (BCMS) 139–141

cloud 23, 94, 107, 122
cloud-based platform 89
cloud-based system 101, 127
Coalition for Epidemic Preparedness Innovations (CEPI) 54, 56

cold chain management 61
collectivism 74–75, 78
compliance 18, 45, 57–58, 66, 72, 76, 89–90, 92, 98, 102, 106, 108, 112–113, 123–124, 126–127, 129, 131, 135–136, 141–142
contact tracing 17–18, 43, 45–46, 57–58, 64, 71, 92
contactless 24, 88, 92, 94, 182
contingency plan (planning) 70, 91–92, 104, 106, 113, 121, 129, 141
corporate social responsibility (CSR) 97–98, 102, 110, 114, 135
COVAX 54, 56–57, 62, 69
crowdsourcing 17
culture 39, 72–80, 86–88, 102–106, 108–110, 112, 116, 120–122, 125, 128, 131–133, 137, 142
curbside 92, 94
curfew 46
customer 21, 23, 90, 92–95, 99–100, 102–106, 108, 112, 114, 118, 121–122, 125, 128–130, 133, 135, 141, 179
customer relationship 90, 130
cybersecurity 24, 53–54, 94, 107–108, 111, 114, 118–119, 127, 182

data analytic 24, 91, 94, 119, 129
death 1–2, 5, 7, *8*, 15, 20, 30, 33, 46, 50, 59, 61, 66, 68, 71, 73, 81–83, **84**, 85–86, 172–177

depression 1, *6*, 11, 23, *28*, 31, 48
digital 3, 12, 16, 23–27, 31, 40–42,
 46, 52–54, 63, 68, 89–95, 97–98,
 100–103, 105, 107–108, 111,
 117–119, 121–122, 127–129, 133,
 141, 181–182, 188–189
digital infrastructure 52, 121,
 128, 141
digital literacy 98, 107, 119, 128, 182
digital payment 24, 52–53, 181–182
digital technology 23, 41, 63, 89, 91,
 94, 117, 129
digital tool 23–24, 26, 46, 53, 119,
 128, 141
digital transformation 3, 23, 25–26,
 40, 52, 54, 63, 89, 92–95, 100,
 102–103, 105, 117, 119, 121–122,
 127–128
digitalization *24*, 53, 91, 111
disinfodemic 38
disinformation 37–38, 50, 58
disparity 32
diversification 91, 99–100, 111, 113

e-commerce 23, 42, 90, 92–95, 100,
 108, 118, 122, 127, 179
e-learning 35, 53, 120
ecosystem 91, 93, 113, 182
education 5, 12, 14–15, 22, 24–27,
 30–31, 33, 35, 52, 62, 65, 68, 69,
 77, 79, 81, 88, 93, 97–98, 110,
 118, 129
educational technology (EdTech)
 26, 93
emergency 1, 4, 6, 13, 57, 61, 68, 89,
 99, 126, 130, 136, 140, 187
employee assistance program (EAP)
 89–90, 95–96, 98, 100, 109,
 131, 135
engagement 18, 27, 55, 58, 65, 90,
 93–94, 97, 100–101, 106, 108,
 110, 114, 118, 125, 127, 135,
 138–139, 141
evacuation 49, 114, 126

facemask 74
factory closure 20

feedback 96, 102, 104, 106, 109,
 110, 115–116, 120, 124, 127–128,
 130–133, 136–138
flexibility 19, 26, 53–54, 69, 89, 93, 96,
 100–102, 105, 107, 109, 121, 129,
 131–132, 138–139, 142, 185
financial stress 29
flexible work arrangement (working
 arrangement) 76, 90, 98, 100–101,
 104, 109, 131, 142
foreclosure 35
furlough 20–21, 29–30, 42, 90, 99

GINI 73, 78–81, **82**, 83, **84**, 85–86
Global Initiative on Sharing All Influenza
 Data (GISAID) 54, 56
governance *6*, 39, 55, 71–72, 74, 104,
 118–119
government support program 90, 100
gross domestic product (GDP) 7–9, 23,
 73, 77–81, **82**, 83, **84**, 85–87
Gross National Happiness (GNH)
 79–80

health declaration 49
health equity 15
health inequality 35
health inequity 15, *16*
healthcare 1–2, 4–6, 14–15, 17–19, 23,
 25, 27, 29–33, 37, 40, 42, 45, 50,
 55, 57–62, 64, 66, 68–69, 71–73,
 77–79, 92, 94, 97, 100, 118, 179,
 188–189
healthcare equity 14–15
healthcare system 2, 4–6, 15, 18,
 30–31, 40, 45, 55, 57–61, 64, 69,
 71–72, 100
herd immunity 18, 56, 61, 68
hospitality 20–21, 30–31, 36, 41, 63, 92
hospitalization 15, 30, 33, 59–62,
 66, *67*
human development index (HDI) 73,
 77–81, **82**, 83, **84**, 85–87
hybrid 25–26, 65, 93, 100–102, 104,
 106–109, 115, 121, 131–132
hygiene 18, 30–31, *47*, 57–58, 60,
 96–97, 114

individualism (IDV) 73, 75–76, 78, 81, **82**, 83, **84–85**, 86–87
inequality 1, 32, *34*, 73, 77, 81, *83*
infection 11, 15, 30–31, 33, 35–36, 43, 48–49, 55, 58, 60–61, 65–67, 72, 141, 168, 180
information sharing 17–18, 37, 54, 56, 70, 72, 77, 79, 91, 142
innovation 2–3, 19, 24, 26–27, 32, 42, 53–54, 89, 92–93, 102–108, 118, 128, 131–134, 179, 182, 188–189
institutional theory (perspective) 73, 75–80, 88
inventory management 91, 111, 129
isolation 11, 15, 18, 26–27, 29–31, *38*, 43, *44*, 45–46, 49, 61, 65–66, 117

Jobkeeper Support Plan (Jobkeeper) 51, 184–185

layoff 20–21, 90, 98–99
leave 21, 42, 96
local sourcing 90–91, 93, 117
localized lockdown 65
lockdown 2, 4, 11, 15, 18, 20, 23, 26–27, 29–30, *38*, 40–42, 45–46, *47*, 51, 54, 57–60, 62–65, 69, 71–72, 76, 87, 89, 97, 99, 110, 122
loneliness 27, 29, 66
long-term orientation (LTO) 73, 75, 78–79, 81, **82**, 83, **84–85**, 86–87

mask mandate 46, 60, 64
mask-wearing 18, 30, 45, 57
Measure of Economic Welfare (MEW) 79
medical supplies 6, 18, 36–37, 55, 58, 60, 64, 97, 100, 178
mental health 11–12, 15, 26–27, *28*, 29–32, 35, 48–49, 65–66, 70, 89, 95–98, 100–101, 104, 107–109, 116, 127, 131, 135, 142

Microsoft Teams 23, 137
movement restriction 30, 45–46
mutant 67
mutation 66–67

nearshoring 91, 111, 129

online 11–12, 22–26, 30–31, 35, 42, 46, 52, 63, 68, 72, 88, 90, 92–95, 100, 107–108, 118–120, 122, 139, 171, 177, 179
online learning platform 24, 26, 120
online mode 25, 42
online payment platform 24
online presence 90, 100, 122
online sales 90, 93
online shopping 22, 63, 88, 93–94
online teaching 72
outbreak 4, 8, 16, 18–20, 31, 37, 43, 46, 49, 52, 57, 59–60, 63–64, 67, 73, 163–179

pandemic fatigue 65–66
partnership 16, 53, 56, 68, 92–93, 104, 111–112, 117–118, 126, 128–129, 131, 179
personal protective equipment (PPE) 4, *6*, 15, 17, 37, 55, 60, 89, 96–97
phased rollout 61
Polymerase Chain Reaction (PCR) test 43
power distance (PDI) 73, 75–78, 81, **82**, 83, **84–85**, 86–87
protocol 4, 13, 18, 29, 42–43, *44*, 45, 54–55, 61, 70, 89, 96, 101, 107, 114, 125–127, 134–136, 140
public health 4–5, 11, 13, 15, 17–18, 31, 36, 40, 43, 45–46, 49–50, 55, 57–66, 68–69, 71, 73, 77, 79–81, *83*, 86–88, 98, 102, 114, 118, 134, 188–189
public health expenditure (HEX) 73, 78–81, **82**, 83, **84**, 85–87
public healthcare 33, 73

quarantine 4, 12, 29, 43, 45–46, 48–49, 55, 64, 71, 76

rapid screening 43
recovery (recoveries) 1, 10, 12, 23, 39–42, 63–64, 73, 81–82, **83–85**, 89, 97, 99, 114, 118, 126–127, 140, 185
reduced working hour 20, 185
remote 2–3, 12, 21, 23–27, 30–31, 33, 35, 40, 42, 52–54, 63, 65–66, 69–70, 75, 89, 92–98, 100–103, 106–109, 114–115, 117–119, 121, 127, 131–132, 135–136, 138, 141–142, 188
remote learning 25–27, 33, 35, 65–66, 93, 97
remote work (remote working) 2–3, 21, 23–24, 30–31, 33, 40, 42, 52–54, 63, 69–70, 75, 89, 93–96, 98, 100–103, 106–109, 114, 117–119, 121, 127, 131, 136, 138, 141–142
resilience 1–3, 18, 24, 32, 39–41, 63, 65–66, 70, 89–91, 93, 98–99, 102–104, 106, 109–113, 117, 119, 121, 123, 127, 129–130, 132, 140–142
responsiveness 93, 106, 124
retail 15, 20–21, 31, 36, 41, 63, 90, 92, 178–179
risk assessment 89, 91, 111–113, 123–126, 129, 132, 134, 136, 140–141
risk management 89, 100, 104, 106, 111–113, 121, 124–125, 130

safety 22, 37, 57, 61, 68–70, 89–90, 92, 94–96, 98, 101, 110, 114, 122, 125, 142, 182, 185
sanitation 22, 89, 96, 101
scenario planning 70, 89, 91, 100, 104, 111–113, 129, 134
school closure 12, 25–26, 31, 33, 46
shutdown 37, 179
small and medium-sized enterprise (SME) 23, 63

social distancing 18, 20–24, 26–27, 29–31, 42, 45–46, 57, 59–60, 63–65, 69, 74, 76, 89, 96, 101
social media 11, 37–38, 42, 50, 95, 134, 139
socio-economic indicator 73, 76, 78–80, 86–87
stay-at-home order 45
stockpile 18, 91, 112
supplier 90–92, 100, 104, 110–111, 113, 121, 125, 128–131, 135, 141, 188
supply chain 2–3, 6, 16, 20, 23–24, 31, 37, 39, 41, 55, 60, 62–64, 70, 90–91, 93–94, 100, 102, 104, 106, 110–113, 117, 119, 121–123, 127–130, 136, 140–141, 178, 189
sustainable 40, 93, 95, 98, 106, 111, 118, 122, 130

technology 2, 12, 17, 23–27, 31, 33, 41–43, 52–53, 61, 63, 70, 89, 91, 93–94, 100–103, 105–108, 110–113, 117–120, 122, 126, 128–129, 131, 133, 136, 141, 179, 182, 188
telehealth 23, 31, 42, 92, 94
telemedicine 42, 88
testing 1, 4, 13, *16*, 18, 27, 31, 33, *38*, 39, 43, *44*, 45–46, 49, 54–58, 60, 64, 68, 71, 95, 125, 136, 140, 187
testing kit 4
tourism 20–21, 30, 63, 117
training 53, 61, 70, 75, 96, 102, 107, 109–111, 113–114, 116, 120–121, 124–126, 128–129, 131–136, 138–140, 142
travel ban 37, 49
travel restriction 4, 20, 30, 37, 40, 45–46, 49, 55, 57, 59, 64, 87, 110, 119

uncertainty avoidance (UAI) 73, 75–76, 79, 81, **82**, *83*, **84**, 85–87
United Nations 39, 74, 166

vaccination campaign 13, 18, 54, 56, 61–62, 64, 68–69, 141, 188–189
vaccine diplomacy 36–37, 118, 187

vaccine nationalism 36, 57
vaccine rollout 64
variant 17, 19, 41, 49, 59, 62, 65–69
ventilator 6, 17, 18, 37, 40, 58, 60
video conferencing 26, 54, 94, 101,
    107, 137
video conferencing platform 26
violence 11–12, 36, 98
virtual 23–24, 26, 32, 40, 42, 53, 63,
    92–97, 101, 104, 107–109, 115,
    119, 132–133, 135–139

wave 1–2, 58–61, 63–66, 68–70,
    75, 141
WebEx 23
well-being 3, 5, 7, 11, 26–27, 29–30,
    32, 35, 66, 70, 74, 79–81, 90,
    95–98, 100–102, 104, 106–110,
    114, 116, 122, 125, 127, 131–132,
    135, 141
work-from-home (WFH) 23, 46

Zoom 23, 31

For Product Safety Concerns and Information please contact our EU
representative GPSR@taylorandfrancis.com
Taylor & Francis Verlag GmbH, Kaufingerstraße 24, 80331 München, Germany

www.ingramcontent.com/pod-product-compliance
Lightning Source LLC
Chambersburg PA
CBHW060303220326
41598CB00027B/4217

9 781032 129785